Cutaneous Manifestations of Endocrine Diseases

Walter K.H. Krause

Cutaneous Manifestations of Endocrine Diseases

With the cooperation of Nathalie Stutz
Foreword by Serge Jabbour

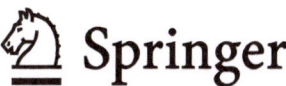 Springer

Em. Prof. Dr. med. Walter K. H. Krause
Philipps-University Marburg
University Hospital
Department of Dermatology
Deutschhausstr. 9
35033 Marburg, Germany

With the cooperation of:
Dr. med. Nathalie Stutz
University Hospital Marburg
Department of Dermatology
Germany

ISBN: 978-3-540-88366-1   e-ISBN: 978-3-540-88367-8

DOI: 10.1007/978-3-540-88367-8

Library of Congress Control Number: 2008936138

Cover design: Frido Steinen-Broo, eStudio Calamar, Spain

Printed on acid-free paper

9 8 7 6 5 4 3 2 1

springer.com

Foreword

Hormones are known to be essential in regulating physiologic processes in each system of the body, including the skin. Endocrine diseases, through excess or deficiencies of hormones, can result in changes in cutaneous function and morphology and lead to a complex symptomatology. Dermatologists may see some of these skin lesions first, either before the endocrinologist, or even after the internist or specialist has missed the right diagnosis. Because some skin lesions might reflect a life-threatening endocrine or metabolic disorder, identifying the underlying disorder is very important, so that patients can receive corrective rather than symptomatic treatment.

In this textbook, "Cutaneous Manifestations of Endocrine Diseases", common and rare endocrine disorders are discussed, with major emphasis on skin manifestations and a brief section on aetiopathogenesis, histopathology and treatment. The list of chapters is exhaustive and offers the dermatologist an excellent overview of the skin lesions resulting from dysfunction of the endocrine system, including diabetes mellitus, obesity, hyper and hypothyroidism, pheochromocytoma, Cushing's, adrenal insufficiency, acromegaly, diabetes insipidus, hyper and hypoparathyroidism, androgen and estrogen excess, pregnancy, and rare syndromes such as carcinoid, glucagonoma, multiple endocrine neoplasia (MEN), autoimmune polyglandular endocrinopathies and other genetic disorders.

Of paramount importance are the chapters on corticosteroids, androgens and estrogens because they constitute the majority of skin-related referrals to dermatologists. Glucocorticoids, either systemic or topical, are commonly used by many physicians to treat a wide variety of medical conditions; long-term use at supraphysiological doses usually induces different cutaneous manifestations, identical to what is seen in endogenous Cushing's. Androgen excess is one of the most frequent problems in women of reproductive age; the main causative disease being polycystic ovary syndrome. In postmenopausal women, it is estrogen deprivation which leads to skin changes. In men, mostly older than 50 years, gynecomastia is a common problem, although these patients will probably not present to the dermatologist unless there are obvious cutaneous signs such as inflammation.

This special and outstanding book is an excellent educational reference for dermatologists and will help them recognize the endocrinopathies causing the various skin lesions they see on a daily basis to provide their patients with the best treatment.

Serge Jabbour, MD, FACP, FACE
Associate Professor of Clinical Medicine
Division of Endocrinology, Diabetes & Metabolic Diseases
Jefferson Medical College, Thomas Jefferson University
Philadelphia, PA 19107, USA

Preface

Skin lesions are important features of many endocrine diseases. Often skin lesions are the first symptom of the disease and lead to the diagnosis. Their description is thus of relevance for early diagnosis and treatment of endocrine disease for specialists in endocrinology as well as in dermatology. Although several skin manifestations of endocrine diseases are illustrative and well-known already to medical students, e.g. Cushing syndrome or acromegaly, in many other diseases the association with endocrine diseases is less clear and self-evident. Mostly, the features are associated with the physiological effects of the hormones to the skin, for the skin is the target organ for a variety of hormones. In endocrine overproduction, the skin lesions are identical as in over dosage of exogenous hormones. In general, skin lesions do not need a special treatment, but their symptoms vary with the intensity of the endocrine disease.

This book describes the clinical and histological features of skin lesions observed in several endocrine diseases. The illustrations show examples of the clinical and histological features. The source of the illustrations is the photo archive of more than 20,000 clinical pictures of the Department of Dermatology, obtained over more than four decades, and a database of a similar number of histological samples. The chapters are arranged according to the order of endocrine diseases in the leading textbook of endocrinology, William's *Textbook of Endocrinology*, thus illustrating the selection of chapters to endocrinologists and enabling them to find descriptions of skin lesions in the diseases they know. The features themselves are described in the language of dermatologists and dermatohistologists to enable the specialists to associate the features observed with the endocrine aetiology. It is a special concern of this book to consider the current scientific literature in the description of aetiopathogenesis and treatment of the cutaneous diseases and to offer the clinician a tool to manage the diseases.

Marburg, 2008   **Walter K.H. Krause**

Contents

List of Abbreviations

AAS	Anabolic-androgenic steroids
ABCD	Asymmetry – border – colouration – diameter
ACTH	Adrenocorticotrophic hormone
AEP	Atopic eruption of pregnancy
AFA	Acromegaloid facial appearance
AGA	Alopecia androgenetica
AIRE	Autoimmune regulator gene
AN	Acanthosis nigricans
APD	Autoimmune progesterone dermatitis
APS	Autoimmune polyendocrinopathy syndrome
APUD	Amine precursor uptake and decarboxylation system
BPH	Benign prostatic hyperplasia
BRCA	Breast cancer gene
cAMP	Cyclic adenosinmonophosphate
CI	Confidence interval
CK	Cytokeratin
CMC	Chronic mucocutaneous candidiasis
CTGF	Connective tissue growth factor
DHEA-(S)	Dehydroepiandrosterone (sulfate)
DI	Diabetes insipidus
DMSO	Dimethylsulfoxide
EGF	Epithelial growth factor
ER	Estrogen receptor
FGF	Fibroblast growth factors
FPHL	Female pattern hair loss
GH	Growth hormone, somatotropin
GnRH	Gonadotropin releasing hormone
G-protein	Guanine nucleotide-binding proteins
HDL-C	High-density lipoprotein
HHV-8	Herpesvirus 8
HRT	Hormone replacement therapy
ICP	Intrahepatic cholestasis of pregnancy
IDDM	Insulin dependent diabetes mellitus
Ig	Immunoglobulin

IGF	Insulin-like growth factors
IHH	Idiopathic hypogonadotropic hypogonadism
IL-2	Interleukin-2
IRS	Insulin-resistance syndrome
LA	Lichen amyloidosus
LCH	Langerhans cell histiocytosis
MC1-R	Melanocortin-1 receptor
MCC	Merkel cell carcinoma
MCV	Merkel cell polyomavirus
MEN	Multiple endocrine neoplasia
MIF	Macrophage migration inhibitory factor
MMAS	Massachusetts Male Aging Study
MMP-1	Matrix metalloproteinases protein 1
MPHL	Male pattern hair loss
MSH	Melanocyte stimulating hormone
NAME	Nevi, atrial myxoma, mucinosis of the skin, endocrine overactivity
NF-1	Neuofibromatosis type I
NFD	Nephrogenic fibrosing dermopathy
NGF	Nerve growth factor
NLD	Necrobiosis lipoidica diabeticorum
NME	Necrolytic migratory erythema
PAI-1	Plasminogen activator inhibitor type 1
PAS	Periodic acid Schiff reagens
PCOS	Polycystic ovary syndrome
PEP	Polymorphic eruption of pregnancy
PF	Pruritic folliculitis of pregnancy
PG	Pemphigus gestationis
POEMS	Polyneuropathy, organomegaly, endocrinopathy, M-protein, skin changes
POMC	Pro-opiomelanocortin
PRKAR1A	Protein kinase A regulatory subunit-1-alpha gene
PSA	Prostate specific antigen
PTH	Parathyroid hormone
PUPPP	Pruritic urticarial papules and plaques of pregnancy
S(HSI)O2	Sum of haemoglobin saturation
SHBG	Sexual hormone binding globulin
SSSS	Staphylococcal scalded skin syndrome
TEN	Toxic epidermal necrolysis
TGF	Tumour growth factor
TIMP-1	Tissue inhibitor of matrix metalloprotease protein
TK-R	Tyrosine kinase receptor
TNF	Tumour necrosis factor
TSH	Thyroid stimulating hormone
UV	Ultraviolett
VEGF	Vascular endothelial growth factor

Posterior Pituitary Hormone, Diabetes Insipidus

1

Synopsis

> Idiopathic diabetes insipidus is rarely connected to specific skin diseases. There are no specific cutaneous manifestations; only singular reports on allergic reactions caused by vasopressin preparations are available.

> Langerhans cell histiocytosis (LCH) is associated in up to 50% of patients with diabetes insipidus. LCH is a clonal accumulation of specific cells resembling normal epidermal Langerhans cells. The skin lesions are agglomerated red or brown papules and tumours with ulceration and incrustation. Diagnosis requires pathohistological investigation, and the singular diagnostic feature is the presence of LCH cells. For treatment, chemotherapy or radiotherapy have been performed.

1.1
Idiopathic Diabetes Insipidus

Aetiopathogenesis. There are two types of diabetes insipidus (DI): central and nephrogenic DI. Central DI is caused by insufficient production of vasopressin, while nephrogenic diabetes insipidus is caused by an impaired response of the kidneys to vasopressin (Majzoub and Srivatsa 2006). The most relevant feature of DI is polyuria. The standard method for diagnosing DI is a water deprivation test; levels of plasma vasopressin should also be measured for differential diagnosis of polyuria. Patients with complete or partial central DI have levels of plasma vasopressin that are subnormal relative to plasma osmolality. In contrast, patients with complete or partial nephrogenic DI or those with primary polydipsia have elevated levels of plasma vasopressin (Sands et al. 2006).

Central DI may be of idiopathic origin, which includes autoimmune diseases or mutations of the arginine vasopressin gene, amounting up to 50% of cases. It may also originate from pituitary tumours such as germinoma or craniopharyngioma, Langerhans' cell

Walter K. H. Krause, *Cutaneous Manifestations of Endocrine Diseases*,
DOI: 10.1007/978-3-540-88367-8, © Springer-Verlag Berlin Heidelberg 2009

histiocytosis (see Section below), and sarcoidosis of the central nervous system as well as from local inflammatory, autoimmune, or vascular diseases, and trauma from surgery or accident (Ghirardello et al. 2005). Traumatic brain injury is followed by severe DI in 2.9% of cases (Tsagarakis et al. 2005; Einaudi and Bondone 2007). The diagnostic method of choice for the cerebral alterations is magnetic resonance imaging (Ghirardello et al. 2007).

Nephrogenic DI may result from hereditary defects of the vasopressin receptor; more than 150 loss-of-function mutations of the vasopressin receptor are known (Thibonnier 2004). Vasopressin acts via the water channels aquaporin 1 (AQP 1) and AQP2, abnormalities of which are demonstrable in nephrogenic DI (Kondo et al. 2006; Schrier 2006). Acquired nephrogenic DI can result from lithium therapy (most common), protein malnutrition, hypercalcemia, or hypokalemia, or may occur after the release of urinary tract obstruction (Sands et al. 2006).

Cutaneous Manifestations. There are no specific cutaneous manifestations of idiopathic diabetes insipidus. However, several unspecific features were observed:

- A case (61-year-old male) has been reported, who showed neither spontaneous nor pilocarpine-induced sweating. Skin histology showed normal eccrine glands. After treatment of DI with desmopressin, normal sweating returned (Shimizu et al. 1997).
- Allergic reactions to treatment for DI, e.g., to deamino-arginine-vasopressin (DDAVP) (Yokota et al. 1982; Itabashi et al. 1982), or cutaneous calcification following injections of depot formulations of vasopressin occurred (Adam et al. 1984).
- DI due to vasopressin antibodies in a patient with systemic lupus erythematosus (SLE) as part of an autoimmune syndrome was observed (Kajiyama et al. 2004).
- DI associated with severe Behcet's disease was observed (Khiari et al. 2003).
- DI associated with or caused by intracranial metastases from mammary carcinoma is a well-known feature (Houck et al. 1970; Tham et al. 1992; Maurer et al. 1993; Yap et al. 1979; Bobilev et al. 2005).

1.2
Langerhans Cell Histocytosis

Aetiopathogenesis. Earlier synonyms for Langerhans cell histiocytosis (LCH) are Abt–Letterer–Siwe disease, Hand–Schüller–Christian disease, eosinophilic granuloma, and histiocytosis X (Nanduri et al. 2000). LCH is a rare disease characterized by the clonal accumulation and/or proliferation of specific dendritic cells resembling normal epidermal Langerhans cells (LCs). An expression of cytokines and cellular adhesion molecules characteristic of LCs has been demonstrated. LCH has a peak age range of 1–3 years in children; it is rare in adults. The specific cells can infiltrate virtually all organs, and most frequently an involvement of bone, lung, skin combined with DI is observed (Makras et al. 2007).

DI has been observed in up to 50% of patients with LCH. Concerning DI in general, one-third of the patients suffer from LCH (Maghnie et al. 2000). Of the patients presenting primarily with DI, 50% will develop also other LCH manifestations within a year. From

11 patients with LCH reported by Kaltsas et al. (2000), 4 four initially presented with DI, but subsequently all 11 developed DI during the course of the disease over a 2-year period. In two large series including 1,741 children and 274 adults with LCH, a 12% and 30% overall prevalence of DI has been found, respectively (Makras et al. 2007). If also hormone deficiencies of the anterior pituitary such as that of the growth hormone, thyroid stimulating hormone (TSH), adrenocorticotropic hormone (ACTH), and gonadotropins were present, the prevalence of DI was still higher, reaching 94%. Isolated anterior pituitary hormone dysfunction without DI has been reported in only 5–20% (Kaltsas et al. 2000). In the study of Nanduri et al. (2000), 50 of 144 patients had one or more hypothalamo-pituitary hormone deficiencies, but 49 of these 50 patients had DI. Isolated DI was additionally present in 29 patients (i.e., in 54.1%). In another study including 125 LCH patients, 10 patients had DI, all of them had concomitant growth hormone deficiency, 4 had impairment of cortisol secretion (two of thyroid hormones and two of gonadotropins) and 4 had hyperprolactinemia (Lin et al. 1998).

Cutaneous Manifestations. The skin lesions are agglomerated red or brown papules and tumours (Fig. 1.1, 1.2). The manifestations may also include crusted dermal areas scattered over the trunk, often healing with depigmentation, and lesions in the perianal region, genitalia, scalp, or behind the ears that often ulcerate. Other areas of manifestation are soft or hard palate, buccal mucosa, tongue, and lips. Cervical, mediastinal, and abdominal lymph nodes may be involved (Makras et al. 2007). The French Langerhans' Cell Histiocytosis Study Group reported skin involvement in 45.8% of 589 patients. The risk for associated pituitary involvement was not increased when compared to patients without skin lesions (Donadieu et al. 2004).

Histopathology. The singular diagnostic feature of LCH is the presence of lesional histoytes (pathological Langerhans cells or "LCH cells"), at least some of which are phaenotypically similar to normal Langerhans cells. There are few reliable markers by which LCH cells from normal Langerhans cells can be definitely distinguished, but Birbeck granules may be one. Birbeck granules are not found in all histiocytes, but only 2–69%. The lesions contain varying proportions of LCH cells, macrophages, lymphocytes, eosinophils, giant cells, neutrophils, and plasma cells. The stage of disease at the time of biopsy is an important factor. There have been no systematic studies of uninvolved lymph nodes in LCH.

In skin lesions, three major reaction patterns have been described (Favara and Jaffe, 1994): a mainly diffuse histiocytic infiltrate pattern that is mainly found in the acute generalized disease (Letterer–Siwe disease), a granulomatous pattern (mainly in the Hand–Schüller–Christian variant), and a xanthomatous pattern (usually found in systemic lesions, rarely in skin lesions). The diffuse histiocytic pattern is characterized by loose aggregates of rather uniform cells in the upper dermis (Fig. 1.3). The cells contain abundant eosinophilic cytoplasm and an infolded or reniform nucleus, sometimes with longitudinal grooves (Fig. 1.4). Epidermotropism may occur focally. The granulomatous pattern consists of sheets and clusters of a polymorphic infiltrate composed of histiocytes, interspersed with eosinophils. Multinucleate giant cells might be prominent. The xanthomatous pattern includes foam cells as well as histiocytes, eosinophils, and multinucleate giant cells.

Immunohistochemically the cells stain positive for S-100-β, CD-1a, and HLA-DR and contain Birbeck granules in electron microscopy (Fig. 1.5).

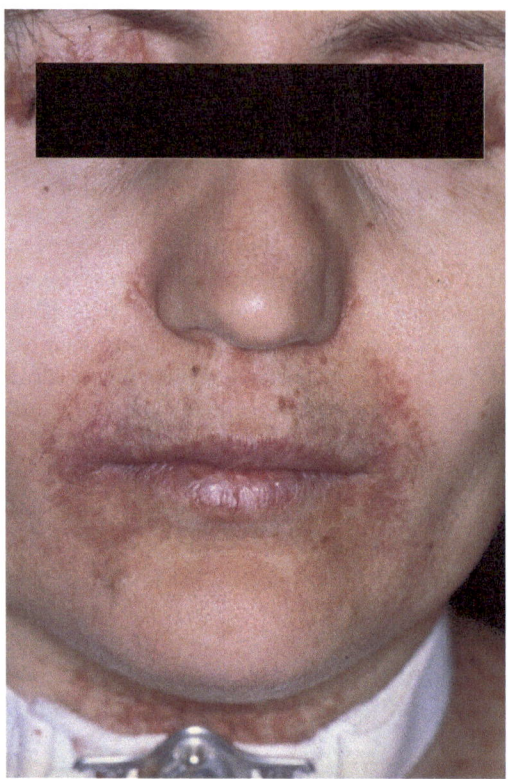

Fig. 1.1 Langerhans cell histiocytosis. The skin lesions are red or brown papules and tumours, which often exulcerate and are covered with crusts. They heal with depigmentation

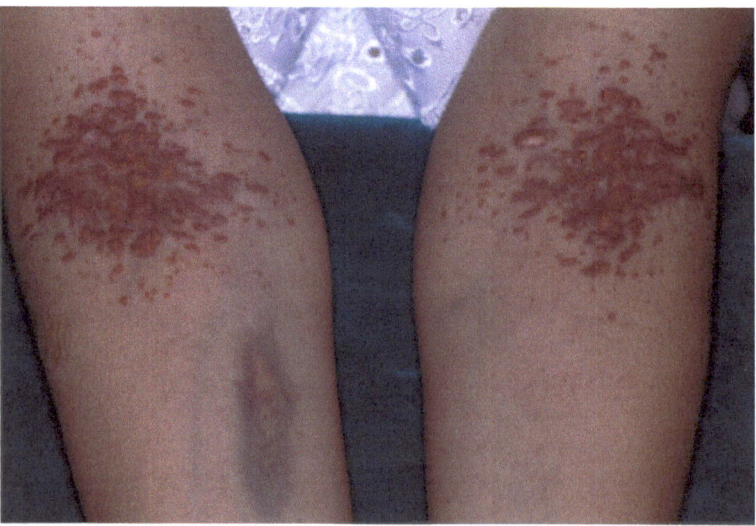

Fig. 1.2 Langerhans cell histiocytosis. Agglomerated red-brownish tumours with intact epidermis

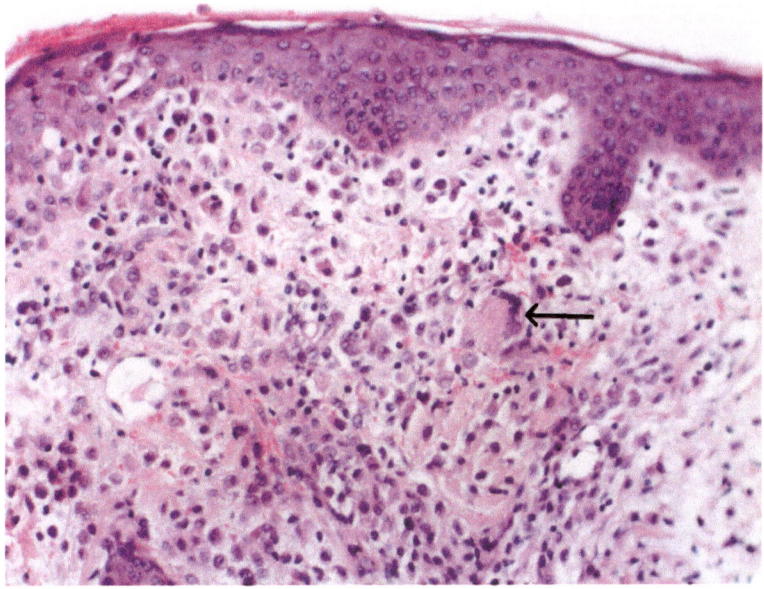

Fig. 1.3 Langerhans cell histiocytosis, histopathology. A diffuse infiltrate of largely histiocytes with abundant eosinophilic cytoplasm and focal epidermotropism and a multinucleate giant cell (*arrow*)

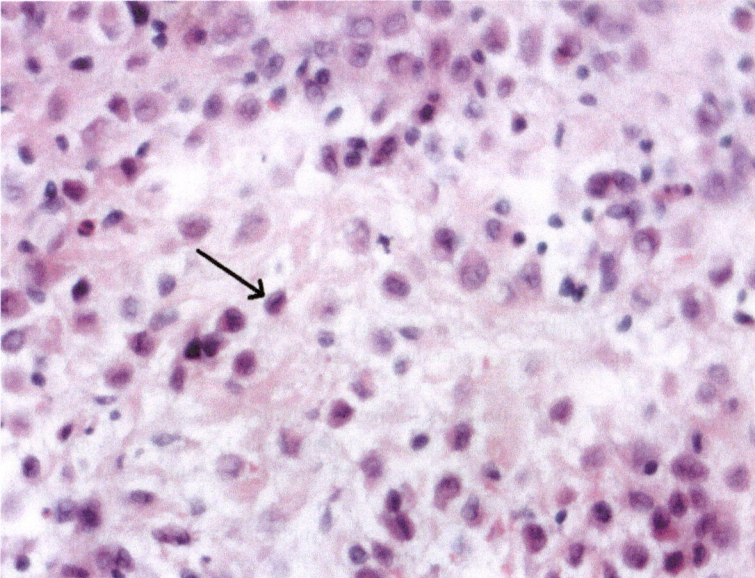

Fig. 1.4 Langerhans cell histiocytosis, histopathology. In a higher magnification, typical reniform or infolded nuclei are visible. In the centre a cell with a longitudinal groove is located (*arrow*)

1

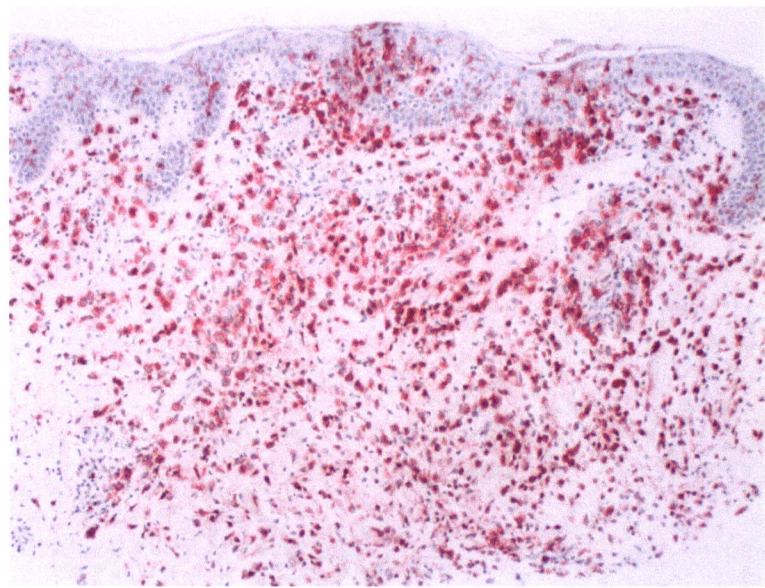

Fig. 1.5 Langerhans cell histiocytosis, histopathology. The LCH-cells stain positive for CD1a

Treatment. There is no standard therapeutic approach to the skin manifestations up to now, in particular because the disease is usually generalized and only exceptionally restricted to the skin. Chemotherapy including the combination of vinblastine with glucocorticoids was the most frequently used (Makras et al. 2007). In addition, radiotherapy was given in a number of cases. Established endocrine deficiencies should be treated with standard hormone replacement regimens. The type of treatment may influence the appearance endocrine abnormalities.

References

Adam A, Rakhit G, Beeton S, Mitchenere P. Extensive subcutaneous calcification following injections of pitressin tannate. Br J Radiol. 1984;57(682):921–2.

Bobilev D, Shelef I, Lavrenkov K, Tokar M, Man S, Baumgarten A, Ariad S. Diabetes insipidus caused by isolated intracranial metatstases in patient with breast cancer. J Neurooncol. 2005;73(1):39–42.

Donadieu J, Rolon MA, Thomas C, Brugieres L, Plantaz D, Emile JF, Frappaz D, David M, Brauner R, Genereau T, Debray D, Cabrol S, Barthez MA, Hoang-Xuan K, Polak M; French LCH Study Group. Endocrine involvement in pediatric-onset Langerhans' cell histiocytosis: a population-based study. J Pediatr. 2004;144(3):344–50.

Einaudi S, Bondone C. The effects of head trauma on hypothalamic-pituitary function in children and adolescents. Curr Opin Pediatr. 2007;19(4):465–70.

Favara BE, Jaffe MB. The histopathology of Langerhans cell histiocytosis. Br J Cancer 1994;70(Suppl 23):S17–S23

Ghirardello S, Garrè ML, Rossi A, Maghnie M. The diagnosis of children with central diabetes insipidus. J Pediatr Endocrinol Metab. 2007;20(3):359–75.

Ghirardello S, Malattia C, Scagnelli P, Maghnie M. Current perspective on the pathogenesis of central diabetes insipidus. J Pediatr Endocrinol Metab. 2005;18(7):631–45.

Houck WA, Olson KB, Horton J. Clinical features of tumor metastasis to the pituitary. Cancer. 1970;26(3):656–9.

Itabashi A, Katayama S, Yamaji T. Hypersensitivity to chlorobutanol in DDAVP solution. Lancet. 1982;1(8263):108.

Kajiyama H, Terai C, De Bellis A, Bizzarro A, Bellastella A, Ohta S, Okamoto H, Uesato M, Hara M, Kamatani N. Vasopressin cell antibodies and central diabetes insipidus in a patient with systemic lupus erythematosus and dermatomyositis. J Rheumatol. 2004;31(6):1218–21.

Kaltsas GA, Powles TB, Evanson J, Plowman PN, Drinkwater JE, Jenkins PJ, Monson JP, Besser GM, Grossman AB. Hypothalamo-pituitary abnormalities in adult patients with langerhans cell histiocytosis: clinical, endocrinological, and radiological features and response to treatment. J Clin Endocrinol Metab. 2000;85(4):1370–6.

Khiari K, Cherif L, Hadj Ali I, Turki S, Lakhoua Y, Ben Abdallah N, Ben Maiz H. Central diabetes insipidus with Behcet disease. A case report. Ann Endocrinol (Paris). 2003;64(6):426–7.

Kondo Y, Morimoto T, Nishio T, Aslanova UF, Nishino M, Farajov EI, Sugawara N, Kumagai N, Ohsaga A, Maruyama Y, Takahashi S. Phylogenetic, ontogenetic, and pathological aspects of the urine-concentrating mechanism. Clin Exp Nephrol. 2006;10(3):165–74.

Lin KD, Lin JD, Hsu HH, Juang JH, Huang MJ, Huang HS. Endocrinological aspects of Langerhans cell histiocytosis complicated with diabetes insipidus. J Endocrinol Invest. 1998;21(7):428–33.

Maghnie M, Cosi G, Genovese E, Manca-Bitti ML, Cohen A, Zecca S, Tinelli C, Gallucci M, Bernasconi S, Boscherini B, Severi F, Arico M. Central diabetes insipidus in children and young adults. N Engl J Med. 2000;343(14):998–1007.

Majzoub JA, Srivatsa A. Diabetes insipidus: clinical and basic aspects. Pediatr Endocrinol Rev. 2006;4 Suppl 1:60–5.

Makras P, Alexandraki KI, Chrousos GP, Grossman AB, Kaltsas GA. Endocrine manifestations in Langerhans cell histiocytosis. Trends Endocrinol Metab. 2007;18(6):252–7.

Maurer J, Busch M, Matthaei D, Helwig A, Duhmke E. Diabetes insipidus und Mammakarzinom –Bedeutung der NMR-Tomografie (MRT) zur Therapieplanung. Strahlenther Onkol. 1993;169(2):126–8.

Nanduri VR, Bareille P, Pritchard J, Stanhope R. Growth and endocrine disorders in multisystem Langerhans' cell histiocytosis. Clin Endocrinol (Oxf). 2000;53(4):509–15.

Sands JM, Bichet DG; American College of Physicians; American Physiological Society. Nephrogenic diabetes insipidus. Ann Intern Med. 2006;144(3):186–94.

Schrier RW. Body water homeostasis: clinical disorders of urinary dilution and concentration. J Am Soc Nephrol. 2006;17(7):1820–32.

Shimizu H, Obi T, Miyajima H. Anhidrosis: an unusual presentation of diabetes insipidus. Neurology 1997;49(6):1708–10.

Tham LC, Millward MJ, Lind MJ, Cantwell BM. Metastatic breast cancer presenting with diabetes insipidus. Acta Oncol. 1992;31(6):679–80.

The French Langerhans' Cell Histiocytosis Study Group. A multicentre retrospective survey of Langerhans' cell histiocytosis: 348 cases observed between 1983 and 1993. Arch Dis Child. 1996;75(1):17–24.

Thibonnier M. Genetics of vasopressin receptors. Curr Hypertens Rep. 2004;6(1):21–6.

Tsagarakis S, Tzanela M, Dimopoulou I. Diabetes insipidus, secondary hypoadrenalism and hypothyroidism after traumatic brain injury: clinical implications. Pituitary 2005;8(3–4):251–4.

Yap HY, Tashima CK, Blumenschein GR, Eckles N. Diabetes insipidus and breast cancer. Arch Intern Med. 1979;139(9):1009–11.

Yokota M, Matsukura S, Kaji H, Taminato T, Fujita T. Allergic reaction to DDAVP (deamino arginin vasopressinin) in diabetes insipidus: successful treatment with its graded doses. Endocrinol Jpn. 1982;29(4):475–7.

Anterior Pituitary Hormones

2

Synopsis

Acromegaly

> Acromegaly results from hyper-secretion of the typical cutaneous manifestations are thickening of the skin and skin folds, of lips and eyelids, and enlargement of the ears and facial bones. The symptoms are reversible with reduction of the hyper-secretion. As a differential diagnosis, several rare acromegaloid-like and hereditary diseases have to be considered.

> Growth hormone as a 'youth hormone' induces similar symptoms, but also more severe symptoms such as hyper-insulinemia, weight gain, carpaltunnel syndrome, increase of intracranial pressure, and enhancement of malignant tumour growth were observed. Because of these side effects, an uncritical use of growth hormone should be urgently discouraged.

Pigmentation Disorders

> α-Melanocyte-stimulating hormone is the main stimulus triggering the activity and morphology of the melanocytes. It is part of the pro-opiomelanocortin (POMC) protein.

> One of its production sites is the pituitary, but a more important source is the skin itself. Diseases of pigmentation in general may be summarized as leukoderma, melanoderma, melanosis, and coeruloderma.

> Endocrine- induced diseases of pigmentation in a narrower sense are Addison's disease (see Chap. 5), and melasma, an acquired hyper-melanosis, occurring on sun-exposed areas of the body.

2.1
Acromegaly

Aetiopathogenesis. The hyper-secretion of growth hormone (GH) induces acromegaly. GH-regulated gene expression contributes to many effects on cellular metabolism, growth, and differentiation. GH regulates physiologically important genes, including those encoding

Walter K. H. Krause, *Cutaneous Manifestations of Endocrine Diseases*,
DOI: 10.1007/978-3-540-88367-8, © Springer-Verlag Berlin Heidelberg 2009

components of the insulin-like growth factors (IGF), axis, and insulin (Quatresooz et al. 2005). They are important in both the development of the organism and the maintenance of normal function of many cells. The system also has powerful anti-apoptotic effects. Specific signalling pathways emanating from the IGF-I receptor affect cancer cell proliferation, adhesion, migration, and cell death (Le Roith and Roberts 2003).

Cutaneous Manifestation. Table 2.1 summarizes the cutaneous features observed in acromegaly (Fig. 2.1). The pasty oedema of the skin is a consequence of an increasing amount of glycosaminoglykans and collagens in the dermis. Also, the water storage is increased because of the increase in hydrophilic compounds of the dermal matrix. The epidermis and the skin appendages become hyper-plastic. Multiple acrochordons (skin tags) develop. Multiple seborrhoic keratoses may occur within a short period, which is often designated as the sign of Leser and Trelart. In earlier publications, the sign was quoted to be associated with malignancies, but this suggestion could not be sustained in more recent papers. The outbreaks of benign skin tumours supports the hypothesis that acrochordons and seborrhoic keratoses are triggered by growth factors (Kilmer et al. 1990; Billon et al. 1996).

The most relevant skin manifestation is enhanced skin thickness. An earlier method for measuring skin thickness was roentgenography (Wright and Joplin, 1969) , which is replaced nowadays by ultrasonography. There was a weak correlation between plasma levels of somatotropin and skin thickness in the patients with acromegaly. Successful treatment of acromegaly (by surgical removal or by radiotherapy of the adenoma) induced decline of skin thickness at a rate of 0.3 mm per year. (Ferguson et al. 1983; Sheppard and Meema 1967). Other simple methods of skin thickness determination used were measurement of hand volume by water displacement (Bhatia et al. 1969) or measuring of a skin fold by a caliper exerting a constant pressure (Harpendon calliper, Fig. 2.2).

Some skin diseases were observed more frequently in acromegalic patients than in normal individuals, including pyoderma gangraenosum and psoriasis. The diseases regressed after treatment of the adenoma. Some authors in the 1970s suggested psoriasis to be a GH-dependent disease (Weber 1984).

Table 2.1 Cutaneous features in acromegaly

Skin	Skin appendages	Pigmentation	Cutaneous vascular reactivity	Skeleton
Thickening, pasty consistency, thickening of skin folds; thickening of lips and eyelids	Widening of follicle ostia, thickening and hardening of the nails, increased secretion of eccrine and apocrine sweat gland, acne inversa, generalized hypertrichosis, bushy eyebrows	Moderate hyper-pigmentation of all skin areas, numerous skin tags	Ischaemia release inducing lower reactive increase in blood flow than in normal individuals. A cold pressure test resulted in a larger vaso-constriction in acromegalic patients.	Growth of bones and cartilages, elongation of the nose, enlargement of the ears, protrusion of zygoma, mandible and chin

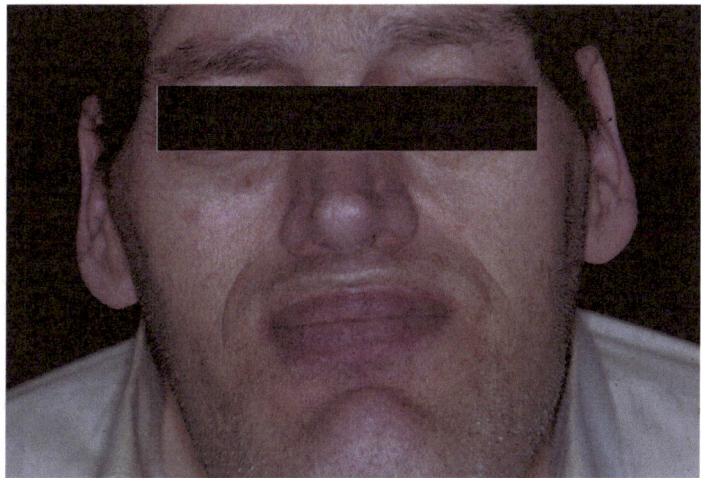

Fig. 2.1 Acromegaly. Typical aspect of the face: the lips and eyelids are thickened, the nose is elongated; zygoma, mandible, and chin are protruded

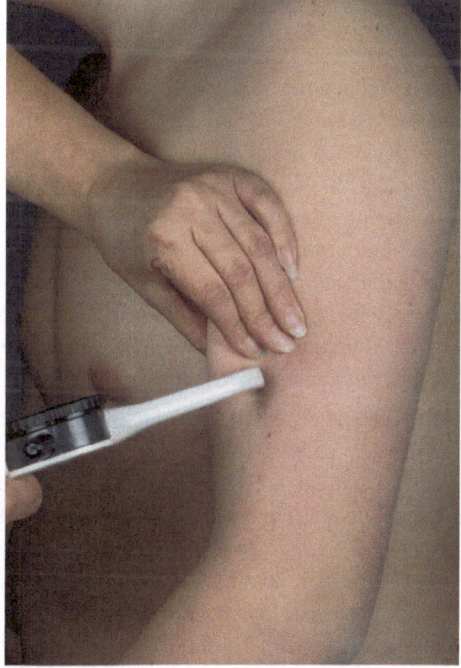

Fig. 2.2 Acromegaly. Measuring of a skin fold by a Harpendon calliper

Sweating in heat and physical stress is reduced. As a consequence of the concomitant hyper-secretion of melanocyte-stimulating hormone (MSH), hyper-pigmentation also occurs.

A special feature is abnormal cutaneous vascular reactivity. Maison et al. (2000) observed cutaneous reactivity in normotensive patients with acromegaly and those with GH deficiency by means of laser Doppler flowmetry at the palms. A warm test induced similar increase in the two groups of patients. Ischaemia release induced lower reactive increase in blood flow in acromegalic patients than in normal individuals. A cold pressure test resulted in a larger vasoconstriction in acromegalic patients. The experiments suggested that the epithelium-dependent vasodilation was impaired, but that the sympathetic-mediated vasoconstriction was increased in acromegaly. Another study (Bach et al. 1992), however, could not show an influence of elevated GH levels in acromegalic patients on cutaneous microcirculation by videomicroscopy of the nail-fold capillaries. Capillary density, torque index, reactive hyperaemia, and epidermal blood flow were not different between patients with normalized GH levels and those with persistently elevated levels.

Several patients with acromegaly-like lesions have been described in the literature. Nguyen and Marks (2003) reported on a patient who was on minoxidil medication for hypertension for more than 10 years. At presentation, he showed an aspect similar to acromegaly. He had longitudinal folds and furrows in the scalp (cutis verticis gyrata) with abundant hair. His earlobes and nose were enlarged markedly and soft, with prominent auricular and nasolabial folds. However, somatotropin and IGF-1 levels were normal. As an explanation the authors quote some data from basic science which support the causative role of minoxidil in the changes observed. In keratinocytes, minoxidil promoted cell proliferation and glycosaminoglycan biosynthesis. In skin fibroblasts, minoxidil stimulated elastin synthesis and increased its messenger RNA level. On the other hand, it decreased collagen production and the secretion of glycosaminoglycan.

Korkij and Plengvidhya (1991) reported on a 39-year-old patient from Thailand with acromegaloid symptoms (thickened nose and lips, enlarged hands and feet, acanthosis nigricans, and multiple skin tags in the axilla, groin, and around the neck) on the basis of Cowdens disease, a dominant inherited disease.

Irvine et al. (1996) described a family with four affected members in three generations, confirming an autosomal dominant pattern of inheritance. In addition to an acromegaloid facial appearance (AFA), they had generalized hyper-trichosis. All other cutanoeus signs of acromegaly and endocrine alterations were absent. Later, Zelante et al. (2000) described a new case of AFA syndrome with an expanded phenotype.

Histopathology. Haematoxylin and eosin (HE) staining of the skin showed slight thinning of the epidermis. The dermis was oedematous, causing separation of collagen fibres leading to a coarsening of collagen bundles. By special staining, the fibres appeared normal both quantitatively and qualitatively. The most consistent abnormality was the observation of dense mucinous deposits in the dermis, consisting from glycosaminoglycan and hyaluronic acid. The increase of skin thickness in acromegaly thus appeared to depend mainly on increased ground substance (Matsuoka et al. 1982).

The extracellular matrix, together with the dermal dendrocytes, was responsible for the mechanical properties of the dermis and the tensegrity. Quatresooz et al. (2005) investigated the structure of the extracellular matrix of the dermis and the number and shape of factor XIIIa-positive dermal dendrocytes in acromegaly. Factor XIIIa is a transglutaminase involved in the deposition and processing of collagen and the arrangement of the cytoskeleton.

Collagen-bundle coarsening and acidic glycosaminoglycan deposits are found irrespective of the current endocrine status and if IGF-1 levels were normalized by treatment. Dermal dendrocytes were often markedly reduced in numbers, but those present were plump with few dendrites (Quatresooz et al. 2005). The skin thickness cannot be taken as a sign of disease activity.

Treatment. A specific treatment of skin lesions is not necessary. They improve, but not always completely, with treatment of the GH hyper-secretion by surgical intervention or radiotherapy of the adenoma. Soft-tissue swelling and facial coarsening improved in continuing treatment in parallel with a decline of growth hormone (Camisa 1989). During treatment with a long-acting somatostatin analogue, patients with acromegaly experienced remarkable improvement in facial features after 0.5–3 months, and the skin became softer, thinner, and paler (Shi et al. 1990). The patients also showed significant reduction in hand swelling after 0.5–2 months of therapy. In half of the patients the shoe size decreased, but not the ring size of the finger.

2.2
Growth Hormone as a Youth Hormone

The secretion of growth hormone declines with age, and the concentration of the insulin-like growth factor, which is produced under the influence of growth hormone, also declines. A substitution of growth hormone in aging individuals therefore appears to be plausible. This was already performed in several studies, and to a certain extent the regulation of dysfunctions was observed. However, often uncontrolled treatment was started without proving a lack of growth hormone secretion. In these cases, the physiological levels were often exceeded, and side effects were observed. These were, particularly in elderly and obese patients, hyper-insulinemia, sodium and water retention, weight gain, oedema in lower extremities, carpaltunnel syndrome, increase of intracranial pressure, papillary oedema, and arthralgies and myalgies. As the most severe side effect, the growth enhancement of malignant tumours was observed (Carroll et al. 1998). All the side effects were reversible after cessation of growth hormone application.

Owing to the side effects described, an uncritical use of growth hormone as a 'youth hormone' should be urgently discouraged.

2.3
Pigmentation Disorders

Aetiopathogenesis. Cutaneous pigmentation is the consequence of two combined events: the synthesis of melanin by melanocytes and the transfer of melanosomes to surrounding keratinocytes. The sequence of processes may be disrupted by different abnormalities of

the molecular events: disorders of melanoblast migration, disorders of melanosome formation, disorders of melanin synthesis in the melanosomes, and disorders of mature melanosome transfer to the tip of the dendrites (Tomita and Suzuki 2004).

Melanins are polymorphous and multifunctional biopolymers, which are photoprotective in human skin and are generally acknowledged as the body''s major defence against
photocarcinogenesis, acting to inhibit the formation of UV-induced DNA photoproducts
(Eller et al. 1996). Human melanocytes produce both the brown–black eumelanin and
reddish–yellow phaeomelanin. Phaeomelanin is the major type in red hair and in the epidermis of skin types I and II. The skin of individuals with dark skin and hair contains large
amounts of eumelanin. It is generally accepted that eumelanin is the more photoprotective
of the two melanins.

Activity and morphology of the melanocytes are triggered mainly by the α-melanocyte-
stimulating hormone (α-MSH). α-MSH is part of the POMC protein, produced
by cleaving of the total protein. One of its production sites is the pituitary, but a more
important source is the skin itself. Melanocytes themselves, keratinocytes, endothelial
cells, and fibroblasts produce POMC protein. Also, human scalp hair follicles possess
a fully functional POMC-MC1 receptor system (Kauser et al. 2005). The POMC production is increased by proinflammatory cytokines, while TGF-β1 negatively regulates
the production. UV exposition exposure enhances the POMC production. A variety of
inflammatory and tumourous skin diseases, in particular those of melanocytic origin,
induce enhanced expression of the POMC system also (Böhm and Luger 2004). The gene
encoding α-MSH is the pro-opiomelanocortin gene. Mutations of the POMC gene
influences the local paracrine, or perhaps autocrine, effects within the epidermis (Tsatmali
et al. 2000; Cui et al. 2007). Melanocytes express also estrogen receptors (ERα and Erβ),
and sex steroids were shown to increase transcription of genes encoding melanogenic
enzymes in normal human melanocytes (Costin and Hearing 2007). This effect is the basis
for the role of natural estrogens and gestagens, pregnancy, and as well as contraceptives in
the pathogenesis of pigmentation disorders.

In addition to the stimulation by α-MSH, melanocytes respond to UV -irradiation,
agouti signalling protein, endothelins, growth factors, cytokines, and other factors. UV
-irradiation also stimulates the production of endothelin-1 (ET-1) and POMC by keratinocytes and those factors also stimulate melanocyte function (Costin and Hearing 2007).

The melanocytes express the melanocortin-1 -receptor (MC1-R), which is activated
by its ligand α-MSH. Adrenocorticotropic hormone (ACTH) is of similar activity as a
ligand of the MC1-R, which activates adenylate cyclase through a G-protein, which in turn
elevates cyclic adenosine monophosphate (cAMP) from adenosine triphosphate. Cyclic
cAMP exerts its effect in part through protein kinase A (PKA) (Tsatmali et al. 2002). The
MC1-R is expressed in nearly all other cell types of the skin such as keratinocytes also of
the eccrine and apocrine glands, endothelial cells, fibroblasts, and mast cells. UV exposition exposure up-regulates the MC1R expression. Specific allelic variants of the MC1
receptor gene are associated with red hair phenotype, melanoma, and non-melanoma skin
cancer. Melanocytes with a non-functional MC1 receptor genes showed an increased
sensitivity to the cytotoxic effects of UV irradiation (Scott et al. 2002).

The biological effects of α-MSH are activation of melanogenesis, resulting in enhanced
skin pigmentation, immune modulation by alteration of cytokin expression, regulation of

secretory activity of the sebaceous glands, regulation of apoptosis of keratinocytes due to oxydative oxidative stress, and the inhibition of collagen synthesis in the dermal fibroblasts (Tsatmali et al. 2002; Böhm and Luger 2004; Artuc et al. 2006). α-MSH promotes the survival of human melanocytes by inhibiting the UV-induced apoptosis independently of the melanin synthesis. If the cells express loss-of-function mutations of the MC-1 receptor, as it is demonstrable in red hair phenotype, this effect is absent, and contributes to the increased tumourigenesis in such individuals. (Kadekaro et al. 2003). In addition to activation of melanin synthesis, α-MSH induces the secretion of a number of cytokins, which are active in operationalizing the effects of sunlight on the skin.

The POMC gene is a p53-responsive gene in keratinocytes, while the response in other cells (melanocytes, fibroblasts) is significantly lower. The identification of p53's transcriptional regulation of POMC/MSH in response to UV thus likely explains the multiple well-described features of the cutaneous pigmentation response. The current findings suggest that, aside from its control of intracellular growth or survival, p53 modulates a secretory pathway that contributes importantly to the physiological response to UV in of skin. For this reason it is perhaps not surprising that a large variety of conditions in human skin may be associated with hyper-pigmentation, including inflammations and tumours (Cui et al. 2007).

Cutaneous Manifestations. Diseases of pigmentation in general may be summarized as follows (Ortonne et al. 2003):

1. Leukoderma (hypopigmentation): resulting from melanocytopenia (lack of melanocytes) or melanopenia (lack of melanin). As a differential diagnosis, non-melanocytic leukoderma has to be considered
2. Melanoderma (epidermal hyper-pigmentation), brown colour: resulting from melanocytosis (increase in number of melanocytes), or melanosis (increase in melanin content of cells)
3. Coeruloderma (dermal hyper-pigmentation), bluish or greyish: melanocytosis and melanophages, melanosis. As a differential diagnosis non-melanotic, e. g. argyria, has to be considered

The tables 2.2, 2.3, 2.4 list some important causes as examples of leukoderma and of epidermal and dermal hyper-melanosis. The diseases will not be described in details herein; the reader may be referred to any competent textbook of dermatology.

Endocrine- induced diseases of pigmentation in a narrower sense are Addison's disease, which is described in the separate Chap. 5, and melasma. Melasma is an acquired hyper-melanosis, occurring symmetrically on sun-exposed areas of the body (Fig. 2.3). The intensity of melasma depends on the skin type and sun exposition; the severity can be clearly diminished by the use of sunscreens. Lesions are irregular, light to dark brown macules and patches, usually involving the forehead, temples, upper lip, and cheeks. Histologically, there is increased amount of melanin in all levels of the cutis, and also the number of melanocytes is increased. The melanocytes appear to be more active in production, but also in transfer of melanin to keratinocytes (Victor et al. 2004).

Treatment. Treatment of melasma is summarized in Table 2.5.

Table 2.2 Diseases with hypopigmentation (from Ortonne et al. 2003)

Etiopathogenesis	Melanocytopenic	Melanopenic
Heritable	Vitiligo (Fig. 2.4)	Albinism
	Piebaldism	
Metabolic		Alpert's syndrome
Endocrine		Hypopituitarism
Chemical	Sulfhydryls	Chloroquine
Nutritional	Vitamin B12-deficiency	Malabsorption
Inflammation	Mycosis fungoides	Pityriasis versicolor var. alba
Neoplastic	Halo nevus	Amelanotic melanoma

Table 2.3 Diseases with epidermal hyper-pigmentation (from Ortonne et al. 2003)

Etiopathogenesis	Melanocytic	Melanotic
Heritable	Lentigines	Café-au-lait macule
	Freckles (Fig. 2.5)	Ephelides
		NAME syndrome
Metabolic		Porphyria cutanea tarda
Endocrine		Addison's disease
Chemical		Arsenicals
Nutritional		Pellagra
Physical		Sun tanning
Inflammation		Post-inflammatory pigmentation
Neoplastic	Melanoma	Mastocytosis

Table 2.4 Diseases with dermal hyper-pigmentation (from Ortonne et al. 2003)

Etiopathogenesis	Melanocytic	Melanotic
Heritable	Mongolian spot	Incontinentia pigmenti
Metabolic		Hemochromatosis
Endocrine		Melasma, dermal (chloasma)
Chemical		Fixed drug eruption
Nutritional		Chronic nutritional deficiency
Physical		Erythema ab igne
Inflammation		Erythema dyschromicum perstans (Ashy dermatosis), Fig. 2.6
Neoplastic	Melanoma	Melanogenuria

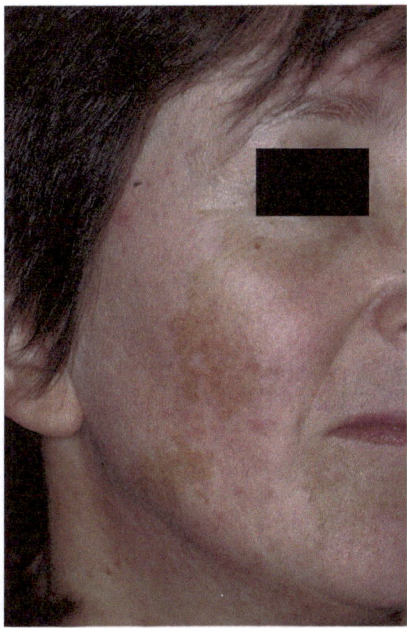

Fig. 2.3 Melasma (chloasma) in a woman. The patchy pigmentation increased in the last 10 years, while the patient used oral contraceptives. The skin shows no alterations besides the pigmentation

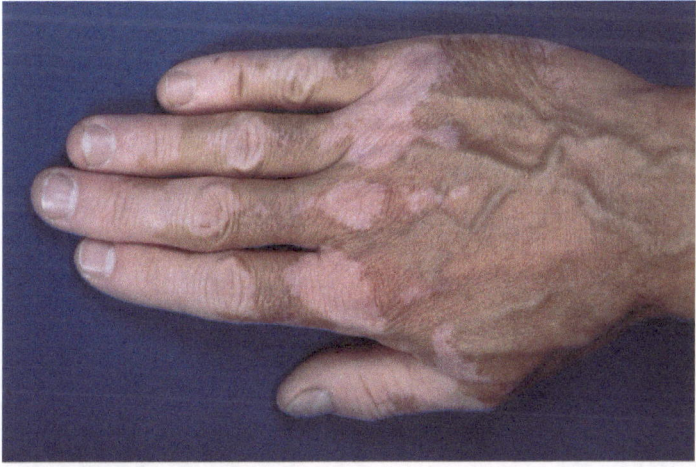

Fig. 2.4 Vitiligo. Hypopigmentation is due to a decrease of number and activity of melanocytes of unknown origin

2

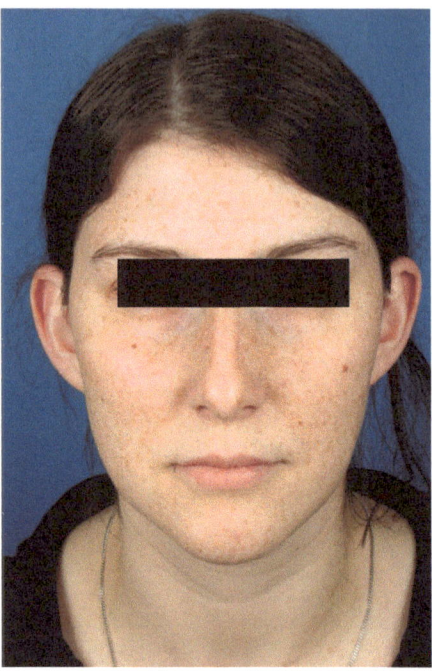

Fig. 2.5 Freckles. Hyper-pigmentation is due to enhanced epidermal activity of melanocytes, increasing with sun exposure

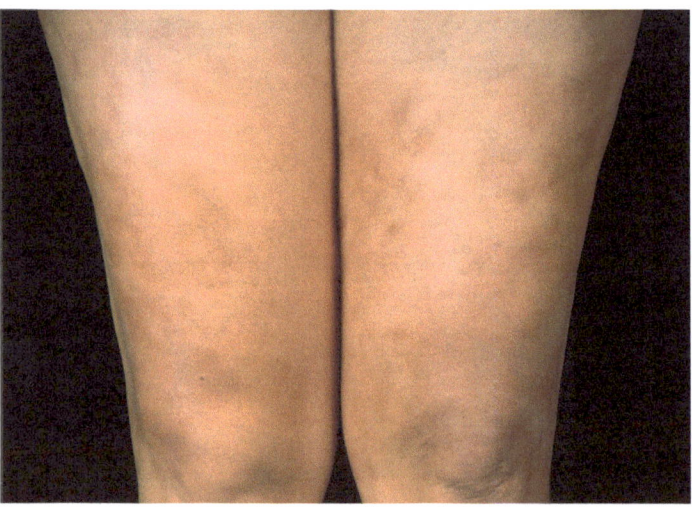

Fig. 2.6 Ashy dermatosis. Dermal hyper-pigmentation as is a consequence of inflammation

Table 2.5 Treatment of melasma (Victor et al. 2004; Rendon et al. 2006)

Class	Treatment	Mechanism of action	Quality of evidence
Phenolic hypopigmenting agent	Hydroquinone	Inhibits tyrosinase, leading to decreased conversion of dopa to melanin	B
Phenolic hypopigmenting agent	N-acetyl-4-S-cysteaminylphenol	A tyrosinase substrate which when exposed to tyrosinase forms a melanin-like pigment	C
Non-phenolic hypopigmenting agent	Glycolic acid (α-hydroxy acid)	Thins stratum corneum, disperses melanin in basal layer of epidermis, enhances epidermolysis, increases collagen synthesis in the dermis	
Non-phenolic hypopigmenting agent	Kojic acid (produced by fungus *Aspergilline oryzae*)	Inhibitor of tyrosinase	D
Non-phenolic hypopigmenting agent	Azelaic acid (saturated dicarboxylic acid)	Reversible inhibitor of tyrosinase; inhibits mitochondrial respiration	B
Non-phenolic hypopigmenting agent	Tretinoin (retinoid)	Enhances keratinocyte proliferation and increases epidermal cell turnover	B
Non-phenolic hypopigmenting agent	Liquiritin (flavanoid)	Disperses melanin from the skin	D
Chemical peel	Glycolic acid peel	Thins stratum corneum, disperses melanin in basal layer of epidermis, enhances epidermolysis, increases collagen synthesis in the dermis	B, C
Laser	Pulsed CO_2 Laser-laser	resurfacing Resurfacing of epidermis	
Q-switched ruby Laserlaser	Ruby Laserlaser	photothermolysis Photothermolysis of melanosomes	C
Laser	Q-switched alexandrite laser	photothermolysis Photothermolysis of melanosomes	C
Dermabrasion	Rotatory diamond fraise	Abrasion of epidermis and dermis	E

Level and quality of evidence for melasma therapies: B, There is fair evidence to support the use of this procedure; C, There is poor evidence to support the use of the procedure; D, There is fair evidence to support the rejection of the use of the procedure; E, There is good evidence to support the rejection of the use of this procedure

2

References

Artuc M, Bohm M, Grutzkau A, Smorodchenko A, Zuberbier T, Luger T, Henz BM. Human mast cells in the neurohormonal network: expression of POMC, detection of precursor proteases, and evidence for IgE-dependent secretion of alpha-MSH. J Invest Dermatol. 2006 126(9):1976–81.

Bach R, Leicht E, Langer HJ, Hartenstein R, Jung F, Berg G, Schatzer-Klotz D, Bonaventura K, Schieffer H, Weinges KF. Kardiale Funktion und kutane Mikrozirkulation bei Akromegalie. Dtsch Med Wochenschr. 1992 117(13):483–9.

Bhatia SK, Hadden DR, Montgomery DA. Hand volume and skin thickness in a normal population and in acromegaly. Acta Endocrinol (Copenh). 1969 61(3):385–92.

Billon C, Beylot-Barry M, Doutre MS, Latapie JL, Roger P, Beylot C. Cutaneous manifestations of acromegaly: 4 cases. Ann Dermatol Venereol. 1996 123(12):821–3.

Böhm M, Luger TA. Alpha-Melanocyten stimulierendes Hormone. Seine aktuelle Bedeutung für die Dermatologie. Hautarzt. 2004 55(5):436–45.

Camisa C. Somatostatin and a long-acting analogue, octreotide acetate. Relevance to dermatology. Arch Dermatol. 1989 125(3):407–12.

Carroll PV, Christ ER, Bengtsson BA, Carlsson L, Christiansen JS, Clemmons D, Hintz R, Ho K, Laron Z, Sizonenko P, Sonksen PH, Tanaka T, Thorne M. Growth hormone deficiency in adulthood and the effects of growth hormone replacement: a review. Growth Hormone Research Society Scientific Committee. J Clin Endocrinol Metab. 1998 83(2):382–95.

Costin GE, Hearing VJ. Human skin pigmentation: melanocytes modulate skin color in response to stress. FASEB J. 2007 21(4):976–94.

Cui R, Widlund HR, Feige E, Lin JY, Wilensky DL, Igras VE, D'Orazio J, Fung CY, Schanbacher CF, Granter SR, Fisher DE. Central role of p53 in the suntan response and pathologic hyperpigmentation. Cell. 2007 128(5):853–64.

Eller MS, Ostrom K, Gilchrest BA. DNA damage enhances melanogenesis. Proc Natl Acad Sci U S A. 1996 93(3):1087–92.

Ferguson JK, Donald RA, Weston TS, Espiner EA. Skin thickness in patients with acromegaly and Cushing's syndrome and response to treatment. Clin Endocrinol (Oxf). 1983 18(4):347–53.

Irvine AD, Dolan OM, Hadden DR, Stewart FJ, Bingham EA, Nevin NC: An autosomal dominant syndrome of acromegaloid facial appearance and generalised hypertrichosis terminalis. J med Genet 1996 33:972–974

Kadekaro AL, Kanto H, Kavanagh R, Abdel-Malek ZA. Significance of the melanocortin 1 receptor in regulating human melanocyte pigmentation, proliferation, and survival. Ann N Y Acad Sci. 2003 994:359–65.

Kauser S, Thody AJ, Schallreuter KU, Gummer CL, Tobin DJ. A fully functional proopiomelanocortin/melanocortin-1 receptor system regulates the differentiation of human scalp hair follicle melanocytes. Endocrinology. 2005 146(2):532–43.

Kilmer SL, Berman B, Morhenn VB. Eruptive seborrheic keratoses in a young woman with acromegaly. J Am Acad Dermatol. 1990 23(5 Pt 2):991–4.

Korkij W, Plengvidhya CS. Multiple hamartoma syndrome with acromegaloidism. Int J Dermatol. 1991 30(1):48–50.

LeRoith D, Roberts CT Jr. The insulin-like growth factor system and cancer. Cancer Lett. 2003 195(2):127–37.

Maison P, Demolis P, Young J, Schaison G, Giudicelli JF, Chanson P. Vascular reactivity in acromegalic patients: preliminary evidence for regional endothelial dysfunction and increased sympathetic vasoconstriction. Clin Endocrinol (Oxf). 2000 53(4):445–51.

Matsuoka LY, Wortsman J, Kupchella CE, Eng A, Dietrich JE: Histochemical characterisation of the cutaneus involvement of acromegaly. Arch Intern Med 1982 142:1820–1823

Nguyen KH, Marks JG Jr. Pseudoacromegaly induced by the long-term use of minoxidil. J Am Acad Dermatol. 2003 48(6):962–5.

Ortonne JP, Bahardoran P, Fitzpatrick TB, Mosher DB, Hori Y: Hypomelanoses and hypermelanoses. In: Dermatology in General Medicine, 6th Ed., Freedberg IM, Eisen AZ, Wolff K, Austen KF, Goldsmith LA, Katz SI (Eds). McGraw-Hill, New York, 2003

Quatresooz P, Hermanns-Le T, Ciccarelli A, Beckers A, Pierard GE. Tensegrity and type 1 dermal dendrocytes in acromegaly. Eur J Clin Invest. 2005 35(2):133–9.

Rendon M, Berneburg M, Arellano I, Picardo M. Treatment of melasma. J Am Acad Dermatol. 2006 54(5 Suppl 2):S272–81.

Scott MC, Wakamatsu K, Ito S, Kadekaro AL, Kobayashi N, Groden J, Kavanagh R, Takakuwa T, Virador V, Hearing VJ, Abdel-Malek ZA. Human melanocortin 1 receptor variants, receptor function and melanocyte response to UV radiation. J Cell Sci. 2002 115(Pt 11):2349–55.

Sheppard RH, Meema HE. Skin thickness in endocrine disease. A roentgenographic study. Ann Intern Med. 1967 66(3):531–9.

Shi YF, Harris AG, Zhu XF, Deng JY. Clinical and biochemical effects of incremental doses of the long-acting somatostatin analogue SMS 201–995 in ten acromegalic patients. Clin Endocrinol (Oxf). 1990 32(6):695–705.

Tomita Y, Suzuki T. Genetics of pigmentary disorders. Am J Med Genet C Semin Med Genet. 2004 131C(1):75–81.

Tsatmali M, Ancans J, Yukitake J, Thody AJ. Skin POMC peptides: their actions at the human MC-1 receptor and roles in the tanning response. Pigment Cell Res. 2000 13(Suppl 8):125–9.

Tsatmali M, Ancans J, Thody AJ. Melanocyte function and its control by melanocortin peptides. J Histochem Cytochem. 2002 50(2):125–33.

Victor FC, Gelber J, Rao B. Melasma: a review. J Cutan Med Surg. 2004 8(2):97–102.

Weber G, Frey H, Neidhardt M. Growth hormone levels in psoriasis. Arch Dermatol Res. 1984;276(6):409.

Wright AD, Joplin GF. Skin-fold thickness in normal subjects and in patients with acromegaly and Cushing's syndrome. Acta Endocrinol (Copenh). 1969 60(4):705–11.

Zelante L, Gasparini P, Savoia A, Lomuto M, Pellicano R. A new case of acromegaloid facial appearance (AFA) syndrome with an expanded phenotype. Clin Dysmorphol. 2000 9(3):221–2.

Zelante L, Gasparini P, Savoia A, Lomuto M, Pellicano R. A new case of acromegaloid facial appearance (AFA) syndrome with an expanded phenotype. Clin Dysmorphol. 2000 9(3):221–2.

Thyroid Hormones

3

Synopsis

Myxoedema and Related Disorders

> In myxoedema due to hypothyroidism, the skin is dry, cool, and pale, it is pasty and voluminous, and shows a non-impressible oedema. Histopathologically, the collagen bundles of the dermis are widely separated by large deposits of mucin. Treatment with substitution of the thyroid hormones induces rapid mobilization of the pathologic proteoglycan deposits.

> Scleromyxoedema (lichen myxoedematosus) showing generalized, indurated lichenoid papules is not associated with hypothyroidism, but it shares the proliferation of fibroblasts and deposition of mucin with myxoedema. The aetiology is unknown. Histopathologically, the dermal intercollagen spaces are widened and filled with glycvosaminoglycans. No standard treatment is known, but the most promising is high-dose intravenous immunoglobulin.

> Nephrogenic fibrosing dermopathy occurs in patients with terminal renal insufficiency. It appears to be induced by the deposition of gadolinium, which is used as a paramagnetic contrast agent. The dermopathy is characterized by a painful, pruritic thickened skin with a *woody* texture. Histopathologically, proliferation of fibroblasts and thickened collagen bundles, distributed haphazardly in the dermis and subcutaneous septa, are found. For treatment, plasmapheresis and high doses of glucocorticoids were used.

Hyperthyroidism

> In hyperthyroidism the skin is warm, tender, and wet with a soft turgor, resembling the infantile skin, and often pruritic. The hair growth cycle may be altered. Distal onycholysis (plummer's nails) is a typical feature.

> Pretibial myxoedema similar to that in hypothyreosis occurs in 4.3% of patients with Graves' thyrotoxicosis and in 15% of patients with Graves' ophthalmopathy.

> Several patients with Graves' disease additionally suffer from vitiligo, urticaria, dermographism, angiooedema, and pruritus.

Walter K. H. Krause, *Cutaneous Manifestations of Endocrine Diseases*,
DOI: 10.1007/978-3-540-88367-8, © Springer-Verlag Berlin Heidelberg 2009

3.1
Myxoedema and Related Disorders

3.1.1
Myxoedema

Aetiopathogenesis. Myxoedema may occur in idiopathic hypothyroidism, in Hashimoto thyroiditis (the most frequent cause), and in thyroid cancer (Larsen et al. 2003; Burman and McKinley-Grant 2006). The term is used to describe specific skin lesions as a consequence of the storage of large amounts of proteoglycans, which are also responsible for the yellowish colour, but also to denominate the skin alterations occurring in hypothyroidism in general.

Localized myxoedema occurs also in Grave's disease, so some authors prefer the term 'thyroid dermopathy' (see Sect. 3.2). Patients exhibit high serum levels of thyroid stimulating hormone (TSH) antibodies. The TSH receptors of fibroblasts may be the antigen responsible for the immune process. It is likely that the fibroblasts are stimulated to produce large amounts of glycosaminoglycans via this mechanism (Fatourechi 2005).

Cutaneous manifestations. In myxoedema, the skin is pasty and voluminous and shows a non-impressible oedema, which is not position dependent. The lesions of myxoedema are asymptomatic, and they are mainly of aesthetic relevance. Increased localized myxoedema may progress to elephantiasis or thyroid acropachy. In addition, the skin of a patient with hypothyroidism is dry, cool, and pale. This appearance is the consequence of the reduced core body temperature and the decreased vascular flow and the decreased reaction to heat. Also, the mucous membranes become dry and the tongue becomes fissured. The epidermis is thin, raspy, and hyperkeratotic (shark skin), and it may present as an acquired keratoderma on the palms and soles. The texture of the stratum corneum is altered. The hairs are dry, fragile, and raspy; sometimes localized alopecia or a diffuse effluvium occur. The nails grow slowly and become brittle and striated, and onycholysis has been reported. Wound healing is decelerated (Ai et al. 2003).

The dermatologic manifestations of hypothyroidism may vary depending on the extent and duration of thyroid disease, but the symptoms are non-specific and do not allow diagnosis without estimation of endocrine function (Burman and McKinley-Grant 2006; Ai et al. 2003). The usual localization of myxoedema in the pretibial area may be related to mechanical factors (Fatourechi 2005). A pretibial mucin deposition on the shins resembling myxoedema was observed in three obese patients by Tokuda et al. (2006).

Various additional dermatologic conditions were observed in association with hypothyroidism in Hashimoto's thyroiditis (Table 3.1). The association does not indicate a causative role of hypothyroidism in these diseases.

A summary of the differential diagnosis to the two other diseases mentioned in this chapter (scleromyxoedema and nephrogenic fibrosing dermopathy) is listed in Table 3.2.

Histopathology. The epidermis shows papillomatosis, and acanthosis with hyperkeratosis (Fig. 3.1). The collagen bundles of the mid- and lower dermis are widely separated of by large deposits of mucin, which stains positively with alcian blue. There is often a mild

Table 3.1 Cutaneous conditions that have been observed in association with Hashimoto's thyroiditis (from Ai et al. 2003; O'Donnel et al. 2005)

Acanthosis nigricans
Acral papulokeratotic lesions
Alopecia
Alopecia areata
Alopecia totalis
Diffuse alopecia
Bannayan–Riley–Ruvalcaba syndrome
Chronic mucocutaneous candidiasis
Dermal mucinosis
Dermatitis herpetiformis (atrophic, but not goiterous variant)
Epidermolysis bullosa
Granuloma annulare
Keratosis pilaris
Leprosy
Lichen sclerosus and atrophicus
Melasma
Mid-dermal elastolysis
Morphea
Onycholysis
Primary localized cutaneous amyloidosis
Pustulosis palmoplantaris
Reticular erythematous mucinosis
Vitiligo
Vogt–Koyanagi–Harada syndrome
Urticaria

superficial perivascular infiltrate but no increase in fibroblast numbers, though a few stellate forms are present.

Treatment. A special treatment in addition to that applied for the thyroid dysfunction itself is not necessary, but in severe cases topical glucocorticoids may be helpful, although this treatment does not alter the natural course. About half of the patients achieve complete remission after several years (Fatourechi 2005). After substitution of the thyroid hormones, the pathologic proteoglycan deposits are quickly mobilized again. Some authors have speculated that topical thyroid hormone might improve xerosis, even in patients with euthyroidism (Ai et al. 2003).

3

Table 3.2 Differential diagnosis of myxoedema, scleromyxoedema, and nephrogenic fibrosing dermopathy

	Myxoedema	Scleromyxoedema	Nephrogenic fibrosing dermopathy
Aetiopathogenesis	Lack of thyroid hormone, deposition of proteoglycans	Unknown aetiology. Association with paraproteinemia consisting of immunoglobulin G	Use of gadolinium as a paramagnetic contrast agent in magnetic resonance angiography in patients with renal insufficiency
Cutanous manifestion	Non-impressible oedema	Skin sclerotization and generalized, flesh coloured, indurated lichenoid papules with or without pruritus	Painful, pruritic thickened skin with a 'woody' texture, resembling peau d'orange
Histopathology	Separation of collagen bundles of the mid- and lower dermis by large deposits of glycosaminoglycans (mucin)	Widened dermal intercollagen spaces, filled with gly-cosaminoglycans (mucin). The mucin stains blue in Hale-PAS. Proliferation of dermal fibroblasts	Proliferation of fibroblasts, variable large epitheloid and stellate cells as well as myofibroblasts, thickened collagen bundles, distributed haphazardly. Deposition of insoluble gadolinium in lesional skin has been shown
Treatment	Substitution of thyroid hormone, no local treatment necessary	Most promising was high-dose intravenous immunoglobulin	Improvement after kidney transplantation, plasmapheresis, high doses of gluco-corticoids

3.1.2
Scleromyxoedema

Aetiopathogenesis. Scleromyxoedema (lichen myoedematosus, papular mucinosis) is not associated with hypothyroidism. It shares the proliferation of fibroblasts and deposition of mucin in the dermis with myxoedema, but a thyroid disease is absent. The aetiology is unknown. It is usually associated with paraproteinemia that predominantly consists of immunoglobulin G with κ light chain. Fibroblasts from patients with scleromyxoedema have been found to synthesize a greater quantity of hyaluronic acid than normal fibroblasts and, subsequently, a greater amount of mucin. Several studies have shown that serum from patients with scleromyxoedema and IgG-paraproteinaemia stimulated in vitro proliferation

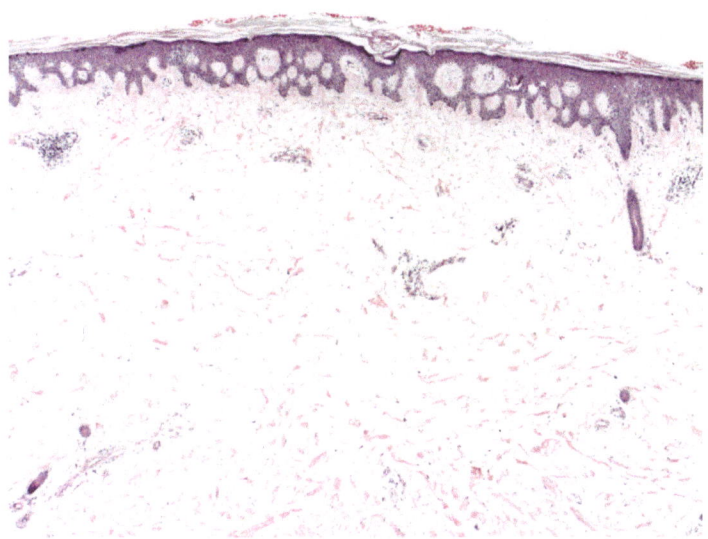

Fig. 3.1 Myxoedema: Papillomatosis, acanthosis, and hyperkeratosis of the epidermis. Large deposits of mucin between collagen bundles in the dermis are seen

of dermal fibroblasts, but a stimulation of fibroblasts by the isolated IgG has not been demonstrated (Kulczycki et al. 2003; Haustein 2005; Georgakis et al. 2006; Lin et al. 2006).

Table 3.2 summarizes the classification and the diagnostic criteria of scleromyxoedema.

Cutaneous manifestation. Scleromyxoedema affects the skin with sclerotization and generalized, flesh-coloured, erythematous or hyper-pigmented, often waxy and indurated lichenoid papules with or without pruritus (Fig. 3.2). Thickening of the eyelids leads to ectropion and lagophthalmus, and hoarseness due to decreased motility of the epiglottis and vocal cords may occur. Also, an enlargement of other hardened body folds is observed (Haustein 2005). As special features, acral papular mucinosis and the discrete papular form were described (Harris et al. 2004; Sulit et al. 2005). Occasionally, the gastrointestinal, cardiovascular, muscular, haematological, and neurological systems are included in the disease (Lin et al. 2006).

Histopathology. Scleromyxoedema is characterized by mucin deposition with a proliferation of fibroblasts in the upper dermis (Lin et al. 2006), but this may be less evident or absent in older lesion. The epidermis shows mild hyperkeratosis and acanthosis, but the surface is flattened (Zakon et al. 1959; Kukova et al. 2006). The dermal fibroblasts show scant or florid proliferation, the dermal intercollagen spaces are widened and filled with glycosaminoglycans, and the collagen bundles are arranged in a whorled pattern (Fig. 3.3). The mucin stains blue in Hale-PAS (Fig. 3.4). A sparse perivascular infiltrate of lymphocytes, occasionally intermixed with eosinophils or mast cells, is present. A decrease of elastic fibres has been reported (Truhan and Roenigk 1986). Ultrastructurally, the fibroblasts are characterized by prominent endoplasmatic reticulum and Golgi apparatus and an increase of mitochondria as a sign for activation and by the presence of

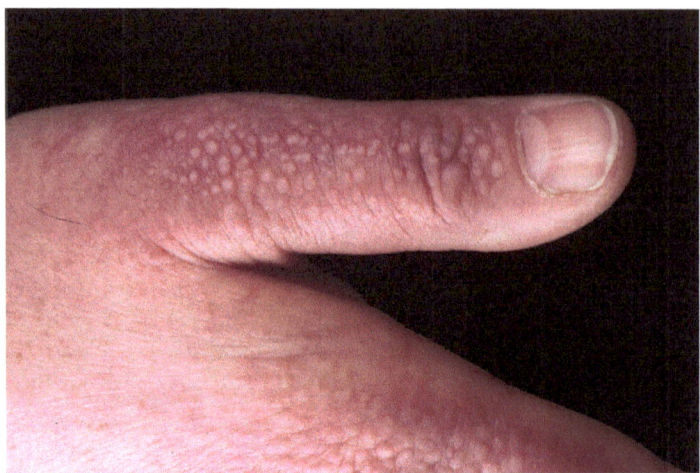

Fig. 3.2 Scleromyxedema. The skin shows sclerotization and long-standing, flesh coloured, erythematous or hyperpigmented, often waxy and indurated lichenoid papules with or without pruritus. This figure illustrates well the former designation "lichen myoedematosus".

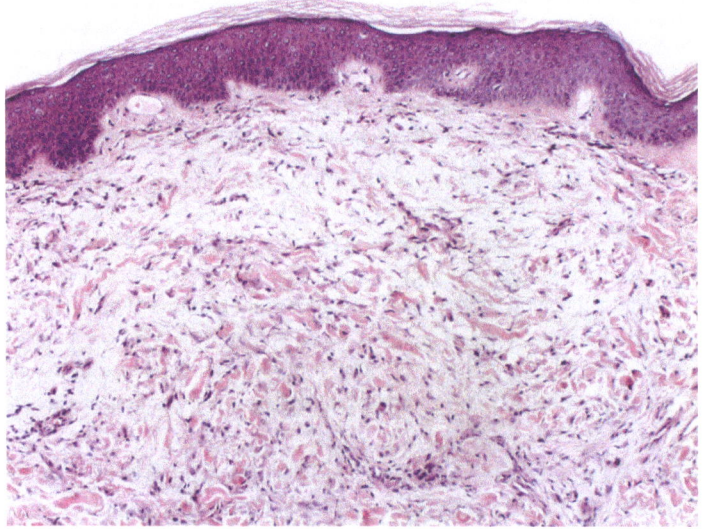

Fig. 3.3 Scleromyxedema: histopathology. Collagen bundles are widely separated by mucin deposits in the upper dermis. The number of fibroblasts is increased

proteoglycanes between the collagen bundles. Numerous dermal spindle (dendritic) cells expressing CD34 and procollagen markers may be interpreted as a CD34+/procollagen population. These fibrocytes may enter sites of inflammation and tissue injury, secrete growth factors and cytokines, and contribute to the matrix production (Haustein 2005).

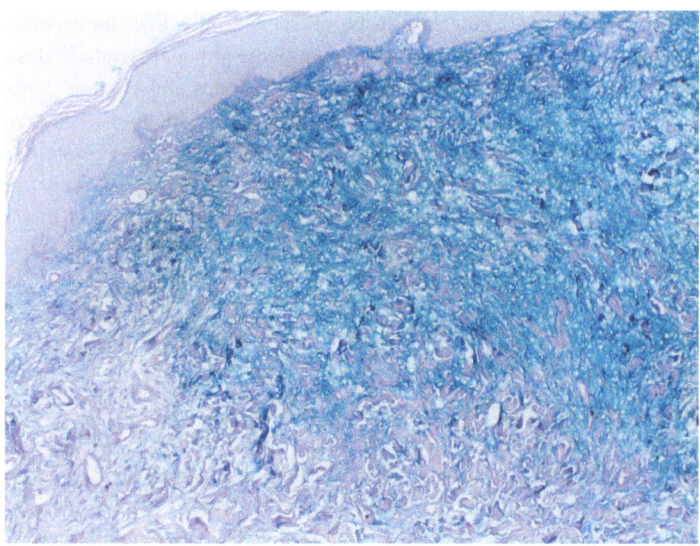

Fig. 3.4 Scleromyxedema: histopathology. The mucin stains blue in Hale-PAS

Table 3.3 Classification and diagnostic criteria of scleromyxedema (papular mucinosis) (Poman and Rudner, 2003)

1. Scleromyxedema
2. Generalized papular and sclerodermoid eruption
a. Microscopic triad: mucin deposition, fibroblast proliferation, fibrosis
b. Monoclonal gammopathy
c. Absence of thyroid disorder
3. Localized lichen myoedematosus
a. Papular eruption (or nodules and/or plaques resulting from confluence of papules)
b. Mucin deposition with variable fibroblast proliferation
c. Absence of monoclonal gammopathy
d. Absence of thyroid disorder
4. Atypical subtypes not fitting the above criteria

The glycosaminoglycan distribution was similar to that found in thyroid diseases or scleroedema (Pomann and Rudner 2003).

Treatment. No standard treatment of scleromyxoedema is known. Trials reported included retinoid, melphalan, corticotrophin, cyclophosphamide, chlorambucil, plasmapheresis, high-dose intravenous immunoglobulin, glucocorticoids (topical, intra-lesional, and systemic), UV-A, extra-corporal phototherapy, and electron beam therapy. However, none of the therapeutic trials appeared to be universally effective. Intravenous immun-globulins appear to be the most promising treatment, although controlled studies are not available (Kulczycki et al. 2003; Lin et al. 2006; Jolles and Hughes 2006; Kukova et al. 2006). As an alternative, thalidomide was introduced in the therapy; a dramatic and prompt improvement in the skin manifestations, reduction of serum paraprotein levels, and decreased mucin deposition and fibroblast proliferation on skin biopsy specimen within a few weeks were observed (Sansbury et al. 2004). The adverse effect of thalidomide is a matter of concern: it induces peripheral neuropathy in 25% of patients and deep vein thrombosis in a considerable number.

3.1.3
Nephrogenic Fibrosing Dermopathy

Aetiopathogenesis. Another important differential diagnosis of myxoedema is nephrogenic fibrosing dermopathy, which was described only in the recent years. It occurs rarely in patients with renal insufficiency. The arguments that gadolinium, which is used as a para-magnetic contrast agent in magnetic resonance angiography, plays an etiologic role are convincing (Bongartz 2007; CDC, 2007; Edward et al. 2007; Grobner and Prischl 2007; Moreno-Romero et al. 2007; Pryor et al. 2007; Kane et al. 2008). An Food and Drug Administration (FDA) warning was published on May 23, 2007, to avoid organic gadolin-ium complexes such as Gadodiamide (marketed as Ominiscan), Gadopentetate dimeglu-mine (GPDG, Omniscan), Gadoteridol (ProHance), and Gadoversetamide (Optimark).

Cutaneous manifestations. Nephrogenic fibrosing dermopathy (NFD) is characterized by a painful, pruritic thickened skin with a 'woody' texture, resembling peau d'orange. The disease first affects the extremities and spreads to the trunk. The flexion of the adjacent joints may be reduced.

Histopathology. In early lesions, a subtle proliferation of fibroblasts and occasionally variable large epitheloid and stellate cells as well as myofibroblasts has been found. The collagen bundles are thickened and distributed haphazardly in the dermis and subcuta-neous septa (Fig. 3.5). There is an augmentation of elastic fibres and in dermal mucin (Cowper et al. 2001). Multi-nucleated histiocytes, sometimes with osteoclast-like mor-phology (Hershko et al. 2004) are present throughout the dermis. CD34+ dermal dentritic cells, CD68+ macrophages, and Factor XIIIa+ cells have been described (Cowper et al. 2001). When the lesions progress, capillary proliferation becomes prominent. In a singular case, calcification of small vessels similar to calciphylaxis has been reported (Edsall et al. 2004). The deposition of insoluble gadolinium in lesional skin was confirmed by X-ray spectroscopy in patients with acute renal failure who underwent magnetic resonance imag-ing with gadolinium (Thakral and Abraham 2007; Kalb et al. 2008).

Treatment. There is no standard treatment of NFD. In some patients the symptoms improved after kidney transplantation. Other patients were successfully treated with plasmapheresis. In addition, high doses of glucocorticoids induced positive responses in a few patients (Haustein 2005).

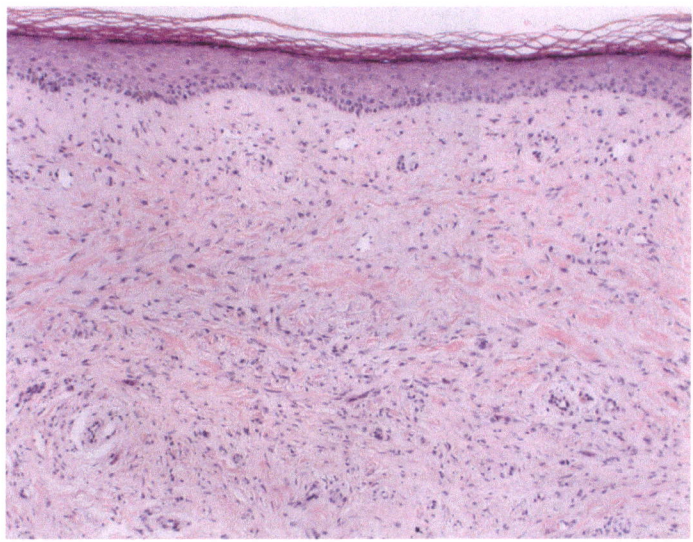

Fig. 3.5 Nephrogenic fibrosing dermopathy: histopathology. Early lesions show a subtle proliferation of fibroblasts and occasionally variable large epitheloid and stellate cells as well as myofibroblasts. The collagen bundles are thickened and distributed haphazardly in the dermis and subcutaneous septa

3.2
Hyperthyroidism

Aetiopathogenesis. Hyperthyroidism may result form autochthonous hyperfunction of the gland or from increased stimulation by the pituitary thyrotropin. The infiltration in thyroid dermopathy (localized pretibial myxoedema) is the consequence of the accumulation of hyaluronic acid in the dermis and the subcutis. The precise pathogenesis of pretibial myxo-edema remains unknown. An autoimmune origin is likely, in which the fibroblasts are stimulated by autoantibodies to thyroid antigens. The predominance in the crural regions is explained by an additional dependent oedema in the lower legs (Fatourechi 2005).

Cutaneous manifestation. In hyperthyroidism the skin is warm, tender, and wet with a soft turgor, resembling to the infantile skin, and often pruritic. It originates from a peripheral vasodilation with increased blood flow, particularly in the face. The patients have a tendency to increased sweating, especially in plantae and palmae. The hairs are thin and tender, and the nails have a normal appearance or are shiny and friable. Also, pigmentation is unaltered. Hair loss or thinning hair can occur in hyperthyroidism, possible due to abecause of an accelerated hair growth cycle. About 5% of patients also develop distal onycholysis with a concave contour (plummer's nails; Fig. 3.6). In men, Graves' disease may be associated with gynecomastia. The mechanism inducing this phenomenon is unknown (Burman and McKinley-Grant 2006).

Fig. 3.6 Distal onycholysis in Graves' disease. The peripheral part of the upper layer of the nail is stripped off from the lower layer (plummer's nails)

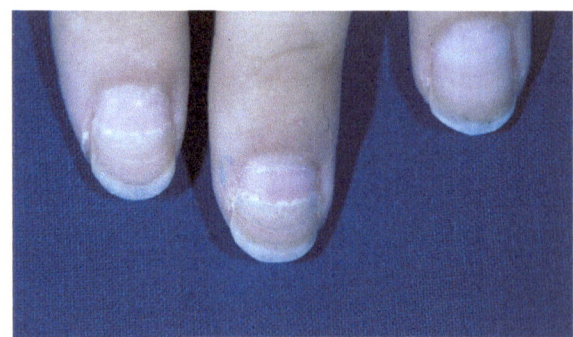

Fig. 3.7 Thyroid dermopathy: The skin is dry and shows a chronic, pasty oedema similar to that in venous insufficiency, which is not position -dependent

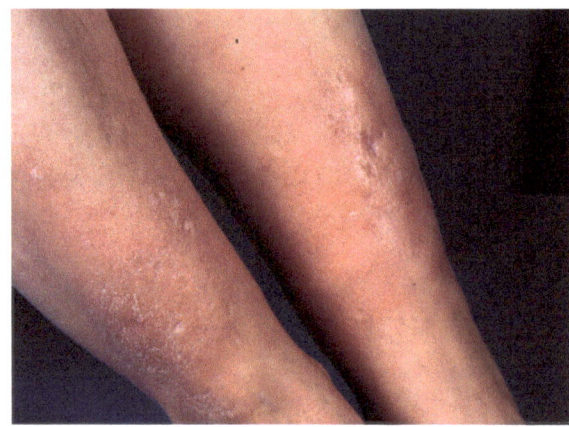

Pretibial myxoedema (thyroid dermopathy) similar to that in hypothyreosis occurs usually bilaterally (Fig. 3.7). Dermopathy was present in 4.3% of patients with Graves' thyrotoxicosis and in 15% of patients with Graves' ophthalmopathy. The lesions show 'peau d'orange' texture and may be hyperkeratotic. Biopsy should be avoided, as the skin does not heal well in this area. Histological investigation is of little use, since only mucin deposits are demonstrable without characteristic alterations (Ai et al. 2003; Burman and McKinley-Grant, 2006). It may arise in other sites, including the hands, arms, shoulders, ankles, ears, and face, and as well as in skin grafts, surgical scars, sport injuries, and animal bites. The most common form is the non-pitting type (58%), followed by nodular forms in 20% and the plaque-like form in 21% of cases.

Several patients with Graves' disease additionally suffer from vitiligo, urticaria, dermographism, angiooedema, and pruritus. However, most of the patients with these diseases are euthyreot.

Treatment. Treatment of localized myxoedema is difficult because normalization of thyroid hormone levels does not always resolve it. Oral steroids, topical steroids with occlusion dressings, intra-lesional steroids, and compression stockings were have been applied tried with limited success. Trials performed in recent years included octreotide, a somatostatin analogue (Ai et al. 2003; Davies and Larsen 2003).

References

Ai J, Leonhardt JM, Heymann WR. Autoimmune thyroid diseases: etiology, pathogenesis, and dermatologic manifestations. J Am Acad Dermatol. 2003;48(5):641–59.

Bongartz G. Imaging in the time of NFD/NSF: do we have to change our routines concerning renal insufficiency? MAGMA. 2007;20(2):57–62.

Burman KD, McKinley-Grant L. Dermatologic aspects of thyroid disease. Clin Dermatol. 2006;24(4):247–55.

Centers for Disease Control and Prevention (CDC). Nephrogenic fibrosing dermopathy associated with exposure to gadolinium-containing contrast agents–St. Louis, Missouri, 2002–2006. MMWR Morb Mortal Wkly Rep. 2007;56(7):137–41.

Cowper SE, Su LD, Bhawan J, Robin HS, LeBoit PE. Nephrogenic fibrosing dermopathy. Am J Dermatopathol 2001;23(5):383–93.

Davies TF, Larsen RP. Thyrotoxicos, pp 374–422. In: Williams Textbook of Endocrinology, 10th Edition, Eds: Larsen PR, Kronenberg HM, Melmed S, Polonsky KS, Saunders, PA 2003.

Edsall LC, English JC 3rd, Teague MW, Patterson JW. Calciphylaxis and metastatic calcification associated with nephrogenic fibrosing dermopathy. J Cutan Pathol 2004;31(3):247–53.

Edward M, Fitzgerald L, Thind C, Leman J, Burden AD. Cutaneous mucinosis associated with dermatomyositis and nephrogenic fibrosing dermopathy: fibroblast hyaluronan synthesis and the effect of patient serum. Br J Dermatol. 2007;156(3):473–9.

Fatourechi V. Pretibial myxedema: pathophysiology and treatment options. Am J Clin Dermatol. 2005;6(5):295–309.

Georgakis CD, Falasca G, Georgakis A, Heymann WR. Scleromyxedema. Clin Dermatol. 2006;24(6):493–7.

Grobner T, Prischl FC. Gadolinium and nephrogenic systemic fibrosis. Kidney Int. 2007;72(3):260–4.

Harris JE, Purcell SM, Griffin TD. Acral persistent papular mucinosis. J Am Acad Dermatol. 2004;51(6):982–8.

Haustein UF. Scleroderma and pseudo-scleroderma: uncommon presentations. Clin Dermatol. 2005;23(5):480–90.

Hershko K, Hull C, Ettefagh L, Nedorost S, Dyson S, Horn T, Gilliam AC. A variant of nephrogenic fibrosing dermopathy with osteoclast-like giant cells: a syndrome of dysregulated matrix remodeling? J Cutan Pathol 2004;31(3):262–5.

Jolles S, Hughes J. Use of IGIV in the treatment of atopic dermatitis, urticaria, scleromyxedema, pyoderma gangrenosum, psoriasis, and pretibial myxedema. Int Immunopharmacol. 2006;6(4):579–91.

Kalb RE, Helm TN, Sperry H, Thakral C, Abraham JL, Kanal E. Gadolinium-induced nephrogenic systemic fibrosis in a patient with an acute and transient kidney injury. Br J Dermatol. 2008;158(3):607–10.

Kane GC, Stanson AW, Kalnicka D, Rosenthal DW, Lee CU, Textor SC, Garovic VD. Comparison between gadolinium and iodine contrast for percutaneous intervention in atherosclerotic renal artery stenosis: clinical outcomes. Nephrol Dial Transplant. 2008;23(4):1233–40.

Kukova G, Bruch-Gerharz D, Gensch K, Ruzicka T, Reifenberger J. Skleromyxödem. Hautarzt. 2006;57(4):326–7.

Kulczycki A, Nelson M, Eisen A, Heffernan M. Scleromyxoedema: treatment of cutaneous and systemic manifestations with high-dose intravenous immunoglobulin. Br J Dermatol. 2003;149(6):1276–81.

Larsen PR, Davies TF, Schlumberger MJ, Hay ID: Thyroid physiology and diagnostci evaluation of patients with thyroid disorders, pp 33–37. In: Williams Textbook of Endocrinology, 10th Edition, Eds: Larsen PR, Kronenberg HM, Melmed S, Polonsky KS, Saunders, PA, 2003.

Lin YC, Wang HC, Shen JL. Scleromyxedema: An experience using treatment witth systemic corticosteroid an review of the published work. J Dermatol. 2006;33(3):207–10.

Moreno-Romero JA, Segura S, Mascaro JM, Cowper SE, Julia M, Poch E, Botey A, Herrero C. Nephrogenic systemic fibrosis: a case series suggesting gadolinium as a possible aetiological factor. Br J Dermatol. 2007; 157:783–787.

O'Donnell BF, Francis DM, Swana GT, Seed PT, Kobza Black A, Greaves MW. Thyroid autoimmunity in chronic urticaria. Br J Dermatol. 2005;153(2):331–5.

Pomann JJ, Rudner EJ. Scleromyxedema revisited. Int J Dermatol. 2003;42(1):31–5.

Pryor JG, Poggioli G, Galaria N, Gust A, Robison J, Samie F, Hanjani NM, Scott GA. Nephrogenic systemic fibrosis: a clinicopathologic study of six cases. J Am Acad Dermatol. 2007;57(1):105–11.

Sansbury JC, Cocuroccia B, Jorizzo JL, Gubinelli E, Gisondi P, Girolomoni G. Treatment of recalcitrant scleromyxedema with thalidomide in 3 patients. J Am Acad Dermatol. 2004;51(1):126–31.

Sulit DJ, Harford R, O'Neill JT. Discrete papular form of lichen myxedematosus: a case report and review of the literature. Cutis. 2005;75(2):105–12.

Thakral C, Abraham JL. Automated scanning electron microscopy and x-ray microanalysis for in situ quantification of gadolinium deposits in skin. J Electron Microsc (Tokyo). 2007;56(5):181–7.

Tokuda Y, Kawachi S, Murata H, Saida T. Chronic obesity lymphoedematous mucinosis: three cases of pretibial mucinosis in obese patients with pitting oedema. Br J Dermatol. 2006;154(1):157–61.

Truhan AP, Roenigk HH Jr. The cutaneous mucinoses. J Am Acad Dermatol. 1986;14(1):1–18.

Zakon SJ, Johnson JH, Grinvalsky H. Lichen myxedematosus (papular mucinosis Dalton and Sidell); report of an additional case. AMA Arch Derm. 1959;79(5):519–23.

Disorders of Calcium Homoeostasis

4

Synopsis

Hypoparathyroidism and Impetigo Herpetiformis

› Impetigo herpetiformis is related to hypoparathyroidism and hypocalcaemia in late pregnancy. Polycyclic oedematous red patches, bordered by tiny pustules in herpetiform distribution start in the flexures and disseminate centripetally. Older patches dry and form colerette-like scales. Histopathologically, intraepidermal Kogoj macropustules originating from migration of neutrophils into higher levels of the epidermis are observed.

› The clinical and histological feature are indistinguishable from those of psoriasis pustulosa. Treatment success with systemic and topical glucocorticoids, ciclosporine, and methotrexate as well as with etretinate has been described.

Hyperparathyroidism

› Hyperparathyroidism may present with generalized pruritus. If patients with secondary hyperparathyreoidism and pruritus in terminal renal insufficiency underwent total parathyroidectomy, pruritus disappeared within few days after surgery.

› Calcinosis cutis designates localized deposits of calcium salts in the skin. They appear as yellow-white, adamant tumours within the skin. Milia-like calcinosis cutis, occurring in patients with Down syndrome, and tumourous calcinosis may be discriminated. Treatment by sodium sulphate or cellulose phosphate and intralesional triamcinolone have been proposed. In some cases, surgical interventions is advisable.

› Calciphylaxis occurs nearly exclusively in secondary hyperparathyroidism in chronic renal insufficiency. It is a life-threatening condition, characterized by livid-reddish and painful necrotic lesions, and localized on finger tips, around the thighs, ankles, buttocks or trunk. They may progress to deep necrotic lesions and heal with massive scarring. In histopathology, deposits of calcium in the walls of subendothelial small blood vessels are visible. As treatment, parathyroidectomy is advisable.

Walter K. H. Krause, *Cutaneous Manifestations of Endocrine Diseases*,
DOI: 10.1007/978-3-540-88367-8, © Springer-Verlag Berlin Heidelberg 2009

4.1
Hypoparathyroidism and Impetigo Herpetiformis

Aetiopathogenesis. Impetigo herpetiformis was first described by Hebra in 1872 in pregnant women. Later, it was related to hypoparathyroidism and hypocalcaemia, occurring mainly in the last trimester of pregnancy, but is was also observed in nonpregnant women and in men (Moynihan and Ruppe 1985). The underlying hypoparathyroidism may be of idiopathic origin (Gueydan et al. 2002) or may occur after surgical removal of the thyroid gland (Moynihan and Ruppe 1985). It occurs also in pregnancy without symptoms of hypoparathyroidism, but patients suffer frequently from compromised general health and hypocalciaemia. The occurrence of impetigo herpetiformis predominantly during pregnancy and its association with hypocalcaemia makes it likely that these factors are relevant in the aetiology of the disease. However, no certain pathological mechanism has been determined so far (Sahin et al. 2002).

Wolf et al. (2005), who observed impetigo herpetiformis in a case with signs of hyperparathyroidism hypothesized that the exsudative inflammation of the skin is the primary event. It may induce a loss of free and protein-bound serum calcium. In order to maintain the calcium homoeostasis compensatory mechanisms are activated, such as stimulation of the parathyroid hormone and mobilization of mineralized calcium from bones. Thus a secondary hyperparathyroidism is induced, which compensates for the loss of calcium. If the compensatory mechanisms are insufficient, hypoparathyroidism may occur.

The incidence of impetigo herpetiformis has not yet been determined. Although its symptoms are quite characteristic, no larger studies but only several of case reports are available in the literature,.

Cutaneous Manifestation. The skin lesions usually start in the flexures and disseminate centripetally. They form polycyclic oedematous red patches, bordered by tiny pustules in herpetiform distribution (Fig. 4.1). The older patches dry and form colerette-like scales (Wolf et al. 2005). Lotem et al. (1989) described the skin lesions as round and polycyclic, oedematous red patches with very small pustules forming a circinate borderline at the periphery. The patches extended centrifugally by new crops of pustules, whereas the older ones dried, giving place to dirty-white scales.

Histopathology. Impetigo herpetiformis is characterized by pustular variants of intraepidermal spongioform (Kogoj) macropustules (Fig. 4.2). The pustules originate from migration of neutrophils from papillary capillaries into higher levels of the epidermis (Fig. 4.3). The keratinocytes in the centre of the pustule become necrotic, and a central cavitation results. The adjacent epidermis becomes thinned with elongated rete ridges. In the dermis, tortuous and dilated capillaries accompanied by a perivascular lymphocytic infiltrate sometimes mixed with neutrophils have been observed (Wolf et al. 2005). Syriou et al. (2005) have described focal liquid degeneration of the basal layer of the epidermis and a moderate lymphocytic infiltrations around the small vessels and fibrinogen deposition in their wall in the dermis. Differential diagnoses include pustular dermatomycosis, bacterial impetigo, candidiasis and pustular drug reactions. For the discrimination of infectious diseases, PAS- and Gram stain are useful, eosinophils indicate drug reactions.

Fig. 4.1 Impetigo herpetiformis. The skin lesions in the flexures form polycyclic edemaous red patches, borderd by tiny pustules in herpetiform distribution. The lesions disseminate centripetally, the older patches dry and form colerette-like scales

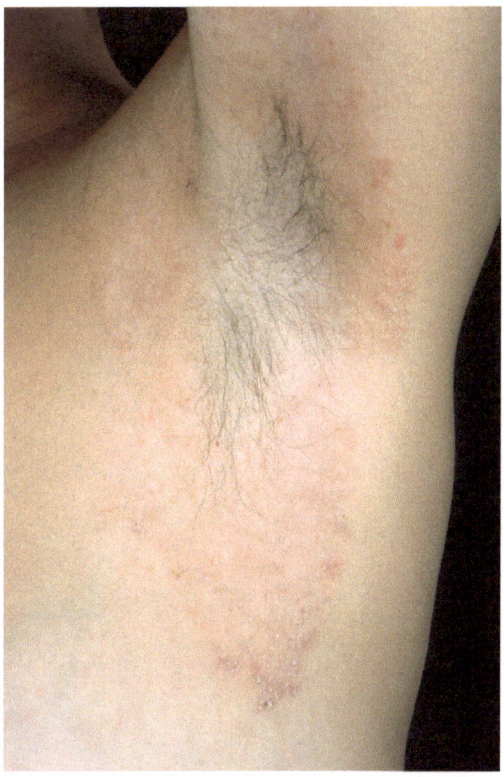

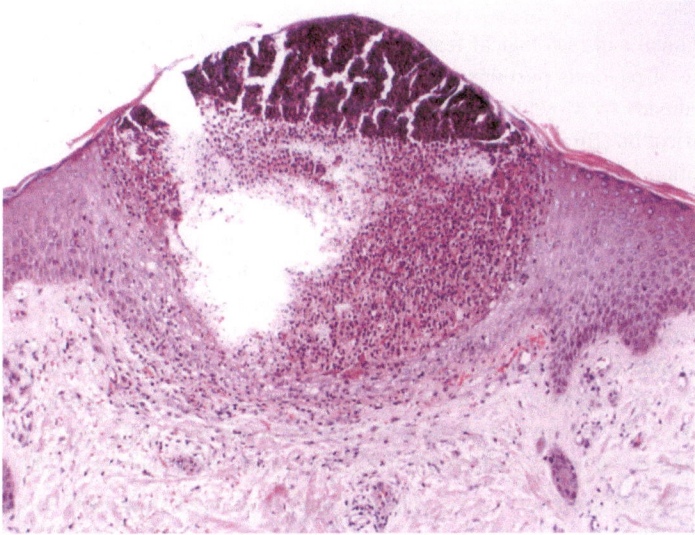

Fig. 4.2 Impetigo herpetiformis, histopathology. View of an intraepidermal macropustules with a scale crust of parakeratosis and neutrophils

Fig. 4.3 Impetigo herpetiformis, histopathology. Upward migration of neutrophils from capillaries in the papillary dermis into the epidermis

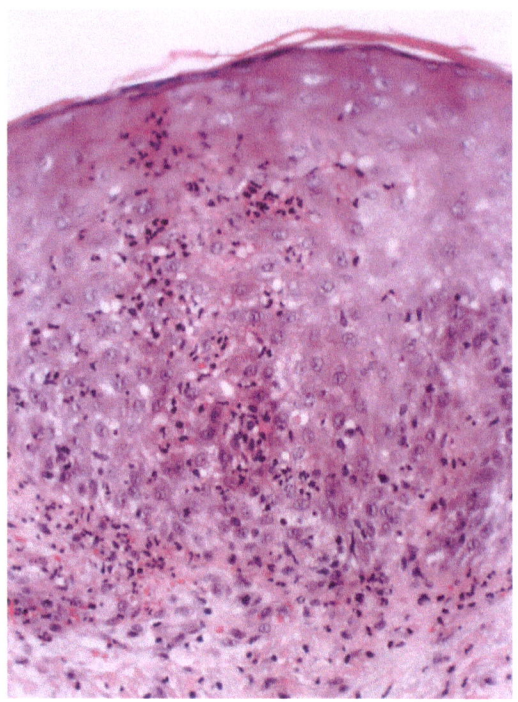

The clinical and histological feature of impetigo herpetiformis are indistinguishable from those of psoriasis pustulosa, and therefore it was considered a variant of pustular psoriasis already by Moynihan and Ruppe (1985). Later, most other authors agreed with this classification (Breier-Maly et al. 1999; Gueydan et al. 2002). As a single report, also an association of hypocalciaemia with a psoriasis-like rash in a nonpregnant individual was described (Syriou et al. 2005). Kuijpers et al. (1997) suggested a common mechanism inducing the features of impetigo herpetiformis and psoriasis pustulosa. In the two diseases, the skin-derived antileucoproteinase, an enzyme that inhibits leukocyte migration in the epidermis, is of lower activity than in plaque psoriasis or in normal skin.

However, other authors have suggested that impetigo herpetiformis is a separate entity. They have pointed out that patients with pustular psoriasis usually have a history of psoriasis, but patients with impetigo herpetiformis have not, and they are free of skin lesions outside the pregnancy. The treatment success with glucocorticoids in pustular psoriasis reveals a striking difference to impetigo herpetiformis (Lotem et al. 1989; Sahin et al. 2002).

Treatment. The treatment of impetigo herpetiformis is not yet standardized. No guidelines have been published to date. Treatment success with systemic and topical glucocorticoids, ciclosporine, and methotrexate as well as with etretinate has been described (Brightman et al. 2007; Bukhari 2004; Lim et al. 2005; Sardy et al. 2006; Valdes et al. 2005).

4.2
Hyperparathyroidism

4.2.1
General Cutaneous Symptoms

Hyperparathyroidism may present with generalized pruritus. Stahle-Backdahl et al. (1989) tested the hypothesis that parathyroid hormone (PTH) is a cause of itching in chronic renal insufficiency. Although patients with pruritus had higher PTH levels than those without pruritus, neither the intracutaneous injection of PTH evoked itching, nor any binding of PTH in the skin was demonstrated by immunohistological methods. The study of Chou et al. (2000), however, suggested a direct influence of Ca_2P on pruritus. Twennty-two of 37 patients with secondary hyperparathyreoidism and pruritus in terminal renal insufficiency underwent total parathyroidectomy and after operation, pruritus disappeared within few days, associated with the normalization of the calcium and phosphorus serum levels. No other factors – PTH level, number of mast cells, levels of IL-2 and TNF-α changed synchronously to the decrease of pruritus.

4.2.2
Calcinosis Cutis

Aetiopathogenesis. Calcinosis cutis designates localized deposits of calcium salts in the skin, usually hydroxyapatite. All skin layers are involved; exceptionally only epidermal and follicular calcifications have been observed without concomitant dermal calcifications (Solomon et al. 1988). Preceding hypercalciaemia is not a condition sine qua non. It occurs idiopathically (Bernardo et al. 1999), as a complication of inflammation, and as a consequence of iatrogenic calcium administration (Arora et al. 2005; Moss et al. 2006). Calcinosis cutis may also be a complication of systemic sclerosis (Meyer et al. 2007). Smack et al. (1996) attempted to classify tumourous calcinosis cutis, which is characterized by juxtaarticular location, progressive enlargement over time, a tendency to recur after surgical removal, and an ability to encase adjacent normal structures. The authors differentiated the following pathogenic mechanisms: idiopathic, primary hyperphosphataemic calcinosis, and calcinosis as a consequence of preexisting diseases, e.g., systemic sclerosis.

Cutaneous manifestations. Calcinosis cutis appears as yellow-white, adamant tumours of different sizes within the skin. Different clinical types are observed: milia-like calcinosis cutis (Fig. 4.4a), which occurs predominantly in patients with Down's syndrome, and tumourous calcinosis (Fig. 4.4b). The pathogenesis of the lesions in individual cases remains unclear (Schepis et al. 1996; Becuwe et al. 2004).

Treatment. There is no specific treatment available (Arora et al. 2005). Fortunately, the course of calcinosis cutis is usually benign. Treatment of calcification of the tissues by sodium sulphate or cellulose phosphate has been proposed. Intralesional triamcinolone acetonide has been shown to reduce the lesions. In some cases, surgical interventions is advisable, and subsequent skin grafting may be required.

Fig. 4.4a Milia-like calcinosis cutis. A number of firm, yellowish, papular lesions are observed at the sole in a child with Down's syndrome

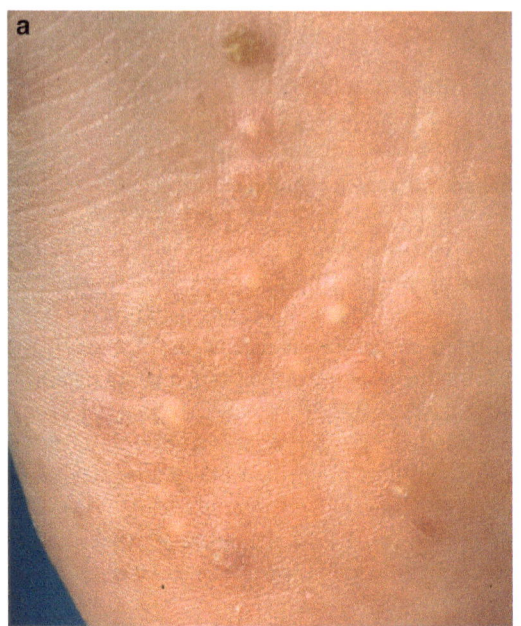

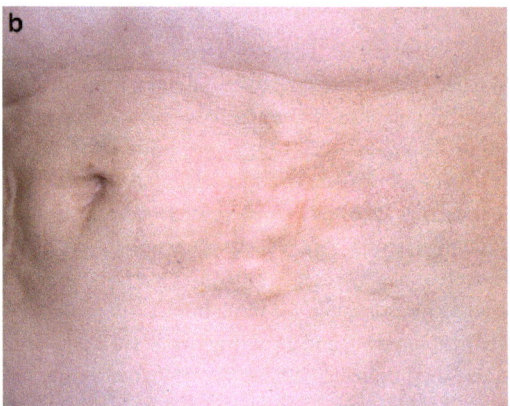

Fig. 4.4b Tumourous calcinosis cutis. On the abdomen, firm, flat tumours are present, which are not relocatable within the skin and can not attributed to cutis or subcutis

4.2.3
Calciphylaxis

Aetiopathogenesis. Calciphylaxis was described as early as in 1962 by Jackson and Munkittrick and in other case reports thereafter (Grosshans et al. 1972; Pulitzer et al. 1990). As synonym, necrotic angiodermatitis (Leray et al. 1995) or calcific–uremic arteriolopathy (Sefer et al. 2001) is found in the literature. Risk factors for the development of calciphylaxis are chronic renal insufficiency, secondary hyperparathyroidism, and hypalbuminaemia (Ketteler et al. 2007). Most descriptions report on patients with chronic renal insufficiency, who develop secondary hyperparathyoidism (Török et al. 1990; Perez-Mijares et al. 1996). There are rare descriptions of patients without renal insufficiency, e.g. by Sefer et al. (2001) of a patient (68 y), who had anticardiolipin antibodies, hyperparathyreoidism and calciphylaxis. She was parathyreoidectomized, the enhanced blood levels of calcium and phosphorus normalized, the anticardiolipin antibodies disappeared, and the necrotic skin lesions healed.

There is evidence that calcification-inhibiting proteins contribute to the pathogenesis of calciphylaxis. Matrix Gla protein, originating from muscle cells of the blood vessels, and fetuin-A from the liver are of particular relevance (Ketteler et al. 2007).

Cutaneous Manifestations. Calciphylaxis is a life-threatening condition in chronic renal insufficiency (James et al. 1999; Wang et al. 2006). It is characterized by livid-reddish and necrotic lesions (Fig. 4.5). The skin lesions are very painful and are localized on finger tips, around the thighs, ankles, buttocks or trunk. They may progress to deep necrotic lesions and heal with massive scarring (Fig. 4.6). The ulcers may be initiated by harmless skin traumata and may undergo secondary infections. It may also appear with the aspect of calcifying panniculitis (Campanelli et al. 2005).

Histopathology. There are deposits of calcium in the walls of subendothelial small blood vessels and within the lumina of medium sized arteries and arterioles in the lower dermis or subcutis combined with hyperplasia of the media (Pulitzer et al. 1990; Török et al. 1990, Fig. 4.7). Occasionally an intimal fibroblastic proliferation and thrombosed vessels as well as massive extravasation of erythrocytes and fat necrosis with a lobular lymphohistiocytic infiltrate has been observed. It is likely that the necrosis and ulceration observed clinically are directly related to vascular occlusion (Lewis et al. 2006).

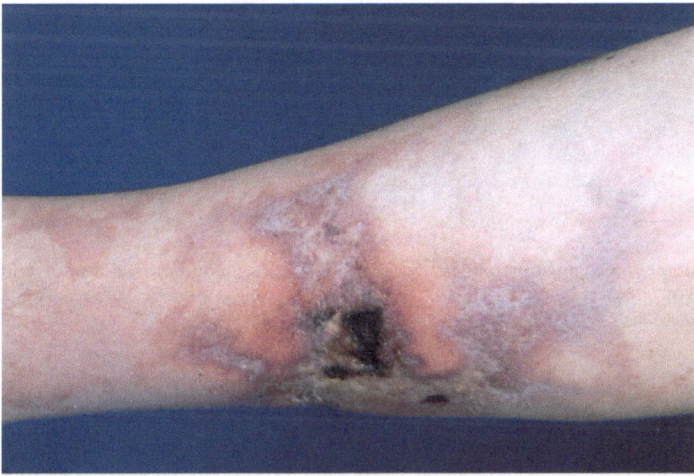

Fig. 4.5 Calciphylaxis is characterized by livid-reddish, painful and necrotic lesions, which may progress to deeply necrotic lesions

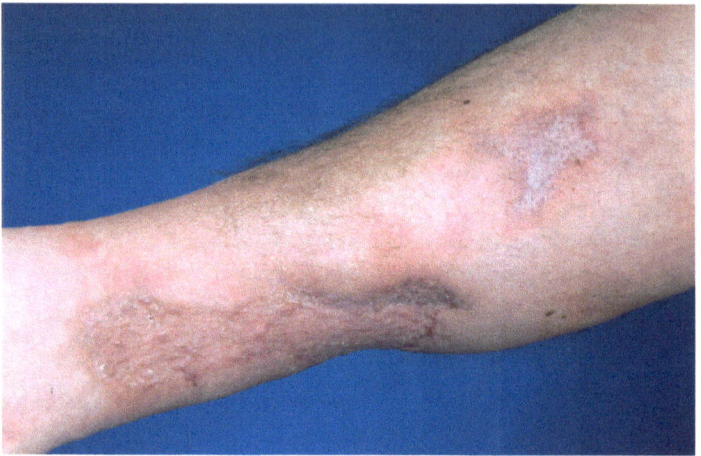

Fig. 4.6 Calciphylaxis. The lesions heal with massive scarring

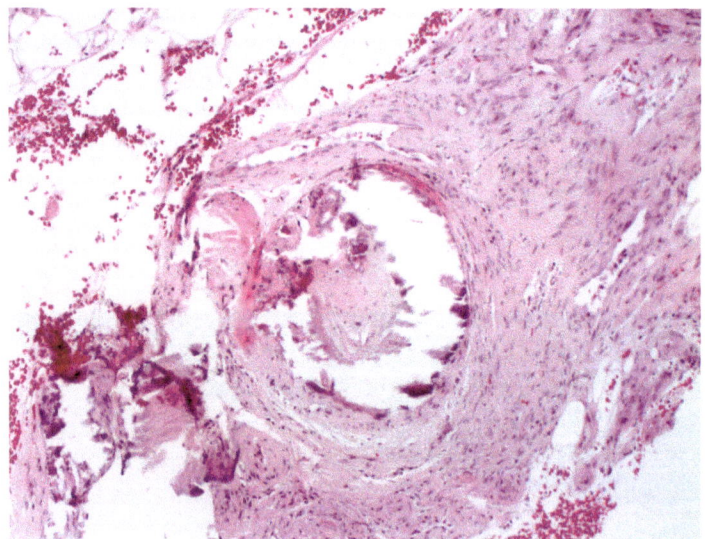

Fig. 4.7 Calciphylaxis, histopathology. Calcification of a medium sized vessel with marked intima proliferation

Treatment. Parathyroidectomy is advisable in severe cases of calciphlylaxis (Tan and Cheong 1996). The patients quoted by Török et al. (1990) and by Sefer et al. (2001) had a benefit from parathyroidectomy. A patient observed in our department being seriously ill for several years of renal dialysis also improved dramatically after parathyroidectomy.

References

Arora A, Agarwal A, Kumar S, Gupta SK. Iatrogenic calcinosis cutis–a rare differential diagnosis of soft-tissue infection in a neonate: a case report. J Orthop Surg (Hong Kong). 2005 13(2):195–8.

Bécuwe C, Roth B, Villedieu MH, Chouvet B, Kanitakis J, Claudy A. Milia-like idiopathic calcinosis cutis. Pediatr Dermatol. 2004 21(4):483–5.

Bernardo BD, Huettner PC, Merritt DF, Ratts VS. Idiopathic calcinosis cutis presenting as labial llesions in children: report o two cases with literature review. J Pediatr Adolesc Gynecol. 1999 12(3):157–60.

Breier-Maly J, Ortel B, Breier F, Schmidt JB, Hönigsmann H. Generalized pustular psoriasis of pregnancy (impetigo herpetiformis). Dermatology. 1999 198(1):61–4.

Brightman L, Stefanato CM, Bhawan J, Phillips TJ. Third-trimester impetigo herpetiformis treated with cyclosporine. J Am Acad Dermatol. 2007 56(2 Suppl):S62–4.

Bukhari IA. Impetigo herpetiformis in a primigravida: successful treatment with etretinate. J Drugs Dermatol. 2004 3(4):449–51.

Campanelli A, Kaya G, Masouyé I, Borradori L. Calcifying panniculitis following subcutaneous injections of nadroparin-calcium in a patient with osteomalacia. Br J Dermatol. 2005 153(3):657–60.

Chou FF, Ho JC, Huang SC, Sheen-Chen SM. A study on pruritus after parathyroidectomy for secondary hyperparathyroidism. J Am Coll Surg. 2000 190(1):65–70.

Grosshans E, Maleville J, Jahn H. Histopathologie und Pathogenese von Calcium-Ablagerungen in der Haut während der Hämodialyse. Z Haut Geschlechtskr. 1972 47(10):467–74.

Gueydan M, Folchetti G, Christofilis MA, Valéro R, Grob JJ, Vialettes B. L'impétigo herpétiforme, un manifestation rare de l'hypocalcémie sévère. Ann Endocrinol (Paris). 2002 63(6 Pt 1):502–4.

Jackson R, Munkittrick R. Secondary hyperparathyroidism in chronic renal disease with metastatic skin calcification. Can Med Assoc J. 1962 87:745–51.

James LR, Lajoie G, Prajapati D, Gan BS, Bargman JM. Calciphylaxis precipitated by ultraviolet light in a patient with end-stage renal disease secondary to systemic lupus erythematosus. Am J Kidney Dis. 1999 34(5):932–6.

Ketteler M, Biggar PH, Brandenburg VM et al. Epidemiologie, Pathophysiologie und Therapie der Calciphylaxie. Dt Ärztebl 2007 104:2959–63

Kuijpers AL, Schalkwijk J, Rulo HF, Peperkamp JJ, van de Kerkhof PC, de Jong EM. Extremely low levels of epidermal skin-derived antileucoproteinase/elafin in a patient with impetigo herpetiformis. Br J Dermatol. 1997 137(1):123–9

Leray H, Dereure O, Canaud B, Teot L, Guilhou JJ, Mion C. Angiodermite nécrotique révélatrice: une hyperparathyrèoidie floride secondaire d'une insuffisance rénale chronique: gérison après parathyroidectomie subtotale. Nephrologie. 1995 16(6):427–30.

Lewis KG, Lester BW, Pan TD, Robinson-Bostom L.0 Nephrogenic fibrosing dermopathy and calciphylaxis with pseudoxanthoma elasticum-like changes. J Cutan Pathol. 2006 33(10): 695–700.

Lim KS, Tang MB, Ng PP. Impetigo herpetiformis–a rare dermatosis of pregnancy associated with prenatal complications. Ann Acad Med Singapore. 2005 34(9):565–8.

Lotem M, Katzenelson V, Rotem A, Hod M, Sandbank M. Impetigo herpetiformis: a variant of pustular psoriasis or a separate entity? J Am Acad Dermatol. 1989 20(2 Pt 2):338–41.

Meyer MF, Daigeler A, Lehnhardt M, Steinau HU, Klein HH. Therapeutic management of acral manifestations of systemic sclerosis. Med Klin (Munich). 2007 102(3):209–18.

Moss J, Syrengelas A, Antaya R, Lazova R. Calcinosis cutis: a complication of intravenous administration of calcium glucanate. J Cutan Pathol. 2006 33 (Suppl 2):60–2.

Moynihan GD, Ruppe JP. Impetigo herpetiformis and hypoparathyroidism. Arch Dermatol. 1985 121(10):1330–1.

Perez-Mijares R, Guzman-Zamudio JL, Payan-Lopez J, Rodriguez-Fernandez A, Gomez-Fernandez P, Almaraz-Jimenez M. Calciphylaxis in a haemodialysis patient: functional protein S deficiency? Nephrol Dial Transplant. 1996 11(9):1856–9.

Pulitzer DR, Martin PC, Collins PC, Reitmeyer WJ. Cutaneous vascular calcification with ulceration in hyperparathyroidism. Arch Pathol Lab Med. 1990 114(5):482–4.

Sahin HG, Sahin HA, Metin A, Zeteroglu S, Ugras S. Recurrent impetigo herpetiformis in a pregnant adolescent: case report. Eur J Obstet Gynecol Reprod Biol. 2002 101(2):201–3.

Sárdy M, Preisz K, Berecz M, Horváth C, Kárpáti S, Horváth A. Methotrexate treatment of recurrent impetigo herpetiformis with hypoparathyroidism. J Eur Acad Dermatol Venereol. 2006 20(6):742–3.

Schepis C, Siragusa M, Palazzo R, Batolo D, Romano C. Milia-like idiopathic calcinosis cutis: an unusual dermatosis associated with Down syndrome. Br J Dermatol. 1996 134(1):143–6.

Sefer S, Trotic R, Degoricija V, Vrsalovic M, Ratkovic-Gusic I, Kes P. Healing of skin necrosis and regression of anticardiolipin antibodies achieved by parathyroidectomy in a dialyzed woman with calcific uremic arteriolopathy. Croat Med J. 2001 42(6):679–82.

Smack D, Norton SA, Fitzpatrick JE. Proposal for a pathogenesis-based classification of tumoral calcinosis. Int J Dermatol. 1996 35(4):265–71.

Solomon AR, Comite SL, Headington JT. Epidermal and follicular calciphylaxis. J Cutan Pathol. 1988 15(5):282–5.

Stahle-Backdahl M, Hagermark O, Lins LE, Torring O, Hilliges M, Johansson O. Experimental and immunohistochemical studies on the possible role of parathyroid hormone in uraemic pruritus. J Intern Med. 1989 225(6):411–5.

Syriou V, Kolitsa A, Pantazi L, Pikazis D. Hypoparathyroidism in a patient presenting with severe myopathy and skin rash. Case report and review of the literature. Hormones (Athens). 2005 4(3):161–4. Review.

Tan HH, Cheong WK. Cutaneous gangrene secondary to metastatic calcification in end stage renal failure—a case report. Singapore Med J. 1996 37(4):438–40.

Török L, Közepessy L, Suhajda K. Unter dem Bild einer kutanen Gangrän erscheinende sekundäre Hyperparathyreose bei einer hämodialysierten Patientin (urämisches Gangrän-Syndrom). Hautarzt. 1990 41(12):689–91.

Valdés E, Núñez T, Pedraza D, Muñoz H. Recurrent Impetigo Herpetiformis: successfully managed with ciclosporine. Report of one case. Rev Med Chil. 2005 133(9):1070–4. Epub 2005 Nov 9.

Wang KL, Li SY, Huang CH, Chen JY. Calciphylaxis. Kidney Int. 2006 70(7):1196.

Wolf Y, Groutz A, Walman I, Luxman D, David MP. Impetigo herpetiformis during pregnancy: case report and review of the literature. Acta Obstet Gynecol Scand. 1995 74(3):229–32.

Wolf R, Tartler U, Stege H, Megahed M, Ruzicka T. Impetigo herpetiformis with hyperparathyroidism. J Eur Acad Dermatol Venereol. 2005 19(6):743–6.

Adrenocortical Hormones

5

Synopsis

Addison Disease

> Addison disease results from a hyposecretion of glucocorticoids in adrenal insufficiency. The most significant feature is generalized skin pigmentation, similar to sun-induced tan.

> The hairs and existing nevi become darker, and the nails show dark bands. Also, hypopigmentation in the form of vitiligo is present in 12% of patients. When the hyposecretion is treated by supplementation of glucocorticoids, the pigmentation resolves.

Cushing Syndrome

> Cushing syndrome occurs as a consequence of hypersecretion of glucocorticoids from the adrenal gland. The most prominent sign is skin atrophy.

> The skin develops a paper-like appearance, becomes thin and translucent, and bruises easily. Also, the typical striae seen on the abdomen, thighs, and arms result from the atrophy.

> The subcutaneous fat increases, leading to the appearance of 'moon facies' and 'buffalo hump'. The cutaneous manifestations resolve with normalization of adrenal hypersecretion.

Drug-Induced Hypercortisolism

> Drug-induced hypercortisolism following application of high doses of systemic glucocorticoids may present with cutaneous manifestations identical to those in Cushing syndrome. Topical application induces adverse effects, which are always more pronounced in the face than in other areas of the body because they are aggravated by sunlight.

> The most common adverse effects are atrophy and the appearance of striae due to a reduction of collagen content. The horny layer barrier is reduced, resulting in increased transepidermal water loss. Wound healing is disturbed. A worsening of cutaneous infections may occur.

Continued

Walter K. H. Krause, *Cutaneous Manifestations of Endocrine Diseases*,
DOI: 10.1007/978-3-540-88367-8, © Springer-Verlag Berlin Heidelberg 2009

5

5.1
Addison Disease

Aetiopathogenesis. Addison disease results from a hyposecretion of glucocorticoids in
adrenal insufficiency, usually due to a primary insufficiency of the adrenal gland following
inflammation or autoimmune diseases. As a consequence, the secretion of POMC from the
pituitary gland increases, which secondarily stimulate melanocyte function (see Sect.
2.2). Addison disease may be associated with other autoimmune diseases, such as lupus
erythematosus, rheumatoid arthritis, diabetes mellitus, or cutaneous autoimmune disorders
(Burke et al. 1986).

Cutaneous Manifestations. The most significant feature of Addison disease is skin pigmentation. The pigmentation is generalized, similar to sun-induced tan (Fig. 5.1), and is

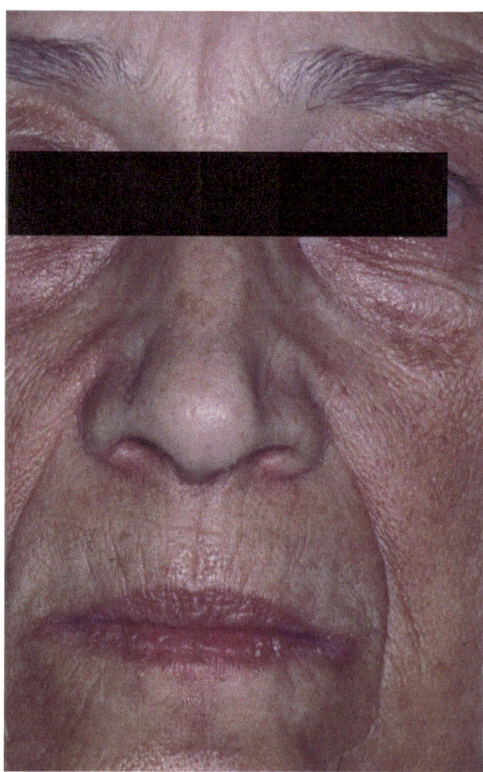

Fig. 5.1 Addison disease. Skin
pigmentation of the face, resembling
sun-induced tan, in a patient with
iatrogenic hyperpituitarism due to
the application of a poorly purified
preparation of adrenocorticotropic
hormone (ACTH)

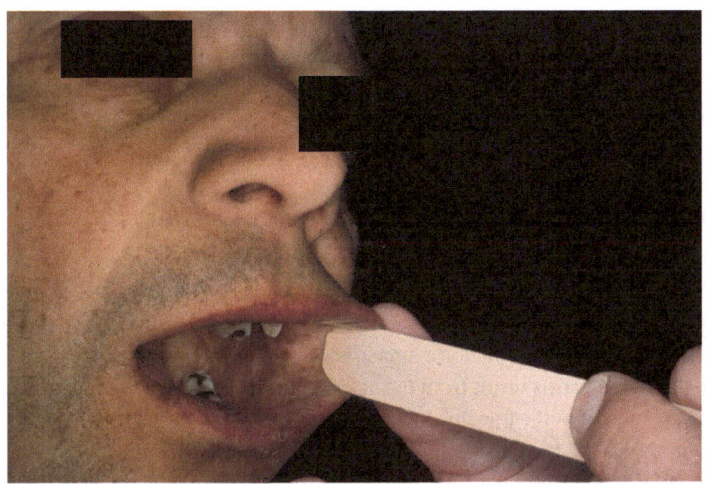

Fig. 5.2 Addison disease. Hyperpigmentation of the oral mucosa (Courtesy of Prof. Althoff, Frankfurt a. M.)

more pronounced in scars, skin folds, hand lines, nipples, perineum, genitalia, and the linea alba (Jabbour, 2003). Sometimes, the pigmentation occurs in the form of freckles. The hairs become darker, and the nails show dark bands. Existing nevi also become darker, and the recognition of the diseases has been facilitated by the computerized image analysis of the nevi, which is thus applicable also as a diagnostic tool in Addison disease (Sunkel et al. 2001). Also, a pathognomonic feature is hyperpigmentation in the oral cavity (Shah et al. 2005; Fig. 5.2). The pigmentation increases slowly with the course of the disease and is often not recognized by the patient himself or will not be considered as a threatening disease, since it will remain the only clinical manifestation for years (Feingold and Elias 1988). The pigmentation may occur before signs of adrenal insufficiency are visible.

Of the patients 12% show a vitiligo. A so-called 'white Addison disease' occurs in rare cases of adrenal insufficiency without skin pigmentation. The mechanism appears to depend on peripheral melanosome degradation of unknown origin, since levels of α-melanocyte-stimulating hormone (α-MSH) are enhanced as typical in these cases (Kendereski et al. 1999).

Treatment. Severe adrenal insufficiency is incompatible with life, and therefore a treatment is mandatory. With sufficient treatment, the pigmentation resolves.

5.2
Cushing Syndrome

Aetiopathogenesis. Cushing syndrome occurs as a consequence of the hypersecretion of glucocorticoids from the adrenal gland. There are primary (adrenal) and secondary (hypophyseal) causes of the hypersecretion. The cutaneous alterations are a consequence of glucocorticoid-mediated suppression of cell proliferation and protein synthesis of keratinocytes as well as dermal fibroblasts, followed by a reduction of the synthesis of skin collagen types I and III as well as other extracellular matrix proteins.

A synchronous hyperproduction of androgens from the adrenal glands often accompanies Cushing syndrome. Women may develop symptoms of female androgenization, the severe virilization was almost exclusively seen in adrenal carcinoma.

In Cushing syndrome due to hypophyseal overactivity, an increased secretion of proopiomelanocortin appears, which may result in hyperpigmentation.

Cutaneous Manifestations. The most prominent sign is skin atrophy. The skin develops a paper-like appearance, becomes thin and translucent, and bruises easily. Ecchymoses occur as a consequence of minor trauma, also after venipuncture. Dilated capillaries appear as telangiectasias, leading to a plethoric appearance in the face. Also, the striae seen on the abdomen, thighs, and arms result from the atrophy (Fig. 5.3). The characteristic purple colour of striae results from the translucency of the skin, which makes the underlying vascular structures more visible (Shibli-Rahhal et al. 2006; Feingold and Elias 1988). In contrast, an increase of subcutaneous fat (centripetal obesity) with weight gain leads to the typical moon facies and buffalo hump (Fig. 5.4). Patients with Cushing syndrome are at increased risk of cutaneous infections by staphylococci, candida, and malassezia species, as well as other fungi, from the immunosuppressive effect of glucocorticoids. Also, infections with

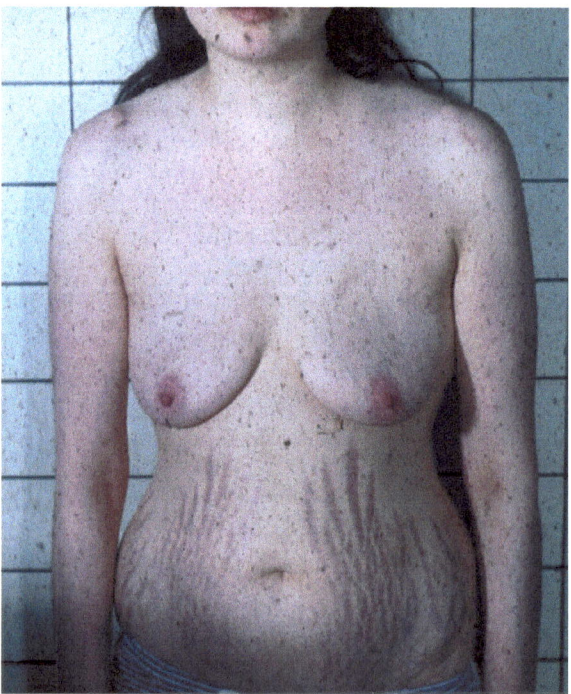

Fig. 5.3 Cushing disease. Dark-red striae distensae in young women, who were on extensive calorie-reduced diet to avoid weight gain (Courtesy of Prof. Althoff, Frankfurt/M.)

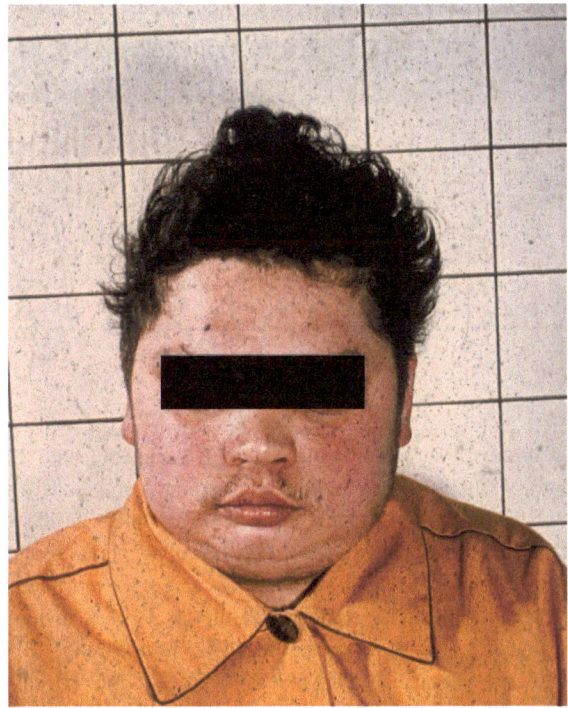

Fig. 5.4 Cushing disease. The increase of subcutaneous fat of the cheeks, resulting in the typical moon facies (Courtesy of Prof. Althoff, Frankfurt/M.)

aspergillus, zygomycosis, or phaeohyphomycosis have been observed. The typical clinical signs are listed in Table 5.1.

Women with Cushing syndrome may develop symptoms of female androgenization: a male-type baldness; excess hair on the face, extremities, and abdomen; vellus hypertrichosis on the upper lip; seborrhoea; and acne. Severe hirsutism, temporal balding, deepening of voice, male body habitus, and clitoral hypertrophy have been observed in adrenal carcinoma (Shibli-Rahhal et al. 2006).

Hyperpigmentation in adrenocorticotropic hormone (ACTH) dependent Cushing syndrome is similar to that in Addison syndrome (Shibli-Rahhal et al. 2006).

With respect to the frequency of the clinical signs among 36 children with Cushing syndrome, Stratakis et al. (1998) quoted purple subcutaneous striae in 28, steroid-induced acne in 21, hirsutism in 14 of 22 girls, acanthosis nigricans in 10, ecchymoses in 10, hyperpigmentation in 6, and fungal infections in 4. No correlation was found between the steroid levels and the severity of the lesions. Intensity of symptoms declined within 3 months after surgical removal of the adrenal tumour, but striae were present in two patients also 18 months post operation.

Cushing syndrome may also include diseases of other organ systems, such as hepatic steatosis, diseases of the gall bladder, pulmonal insufficiency, osteoarthritis, proteinuria, increased haemoglobin concentration, and immune incompetence.

Table 5.1 Clinical features of Cushing syndrome

Epidermis	Dermis	Blood vessels	Skin append-ages	Subcutis
Atrophic, smooth, translucent, defective wound healing	Flaccid, anelastic, vulnerable, defective immune reactions, enhanced risk of infections, dark-red striae distensae	Haematomas, ecchymoses, teleangiectasias, plethora	Increasing vellus hairs, general hypertrichosis, frontal alopecia, altered pigmentation, acne, and hirsutism	Increase of subcutaneous fat (centripetal obesity), weight gain, moon facies, buffalo hump

Histopathology. A histopathological investigation of the skin is of little use. Skin atrophy manifests by thinning of the epidermis and flattening of the dermoepidermal junction with a concomitant decrease in dermal ground substance. The inter-fibrillar spaces between collagen and elastin collapse, and reorientation of the collagen and elastin fibres follows (Groves et al. 1990). A study has suggested that this stage is characterized by mast cell degranulation followed by elastophagocytosis (Sheu et al. 1991). The biochemical determination of collagen content has shown values below the normal range (Black et al. 1973). In late lesions, an increase and thickening of elastic fibres in the reticular dermis and an increase in glycosaminoglycanes in the dermis of striae distensae have been described (Watson et al. 1998).

Treatment. The cutaneous manifestations resolve with normalization of adrenal hypersecretion. Striae distensae become pale, but remain visible.

5.3
Drug-Induced Hypercortisolism

Aetiopathogenesis. The long-term application of glucocorticoids at a dose exceeding the daily production of endogenous cortisol (more than 20 mg) usually induces cutaneous manifestations identical to the endogenous hypersecretion in Cushing syndrome. The clinical appearance is indistinguishable without data on the medical history.

The most relevant adverse effect of glucocorticoid therapy is atrophy of the skin (see below). It is mainly caused by suppression of cutaneous cell proliferation and protein synthesis, which concerns keratinocytes as well as dermal fibroblasts (Schäcke et al. 2002). The synthesis of skin collagen types I and III was found to be reduced by 39–63% after inhalation of budesonide. Glucocorticoids reduce the proliferative activity of keratinocytes and dermal fibroblasts, resulting in depressed collagen turnover. A decrease of collagen I and III synthesis has been demonstrated at both mRNA and protein levels. Also, a depression of other extracellular matrix proteins occurs. Similarly, elastin synthesis is significantly down-regulated by hydrocortisone in vitro. Additionally, glucocorticoids intervene in the regulation of pro-inflammatory cytokines, growth factors, matrix proteins, and matrix proteases, which have impact on wound healing (Schäcke et al. 2002).

Adverse effects of glucocorticoid therapy are usually more severe after systemic rather than topical application. An ideal topical glucocorticoid should permeate well through the stratum corneum and penetrate into the skin but should not lead to enhanced concentrations in the blood serum. However, topically administered glucocorticoids may be followed by systemic reactions due to the rapid resorption of the drug through the skin such as in drug-induced Cushing syndrome, osteopathy, and metabolic glucose intolerance. Children are more prone to develop systemic reactions to topically applied medication because of their higher ratio of total body surface area to body weight. The structure and composition of the skin itself, however, are not clearly different from those of adults (Hengge et al. 2006). Adverse effect to the skin occurs also in patients taking high-dose inhaled glucocorticoids (Hanania et al. 1995). This risk increases with age, dose, and duration of inhalation therapy.

The adverse effects are in principle inseparably connected to the anti-inflammatory effects of glucocorticoids. Glucocorticoids bind to the glucocorticoid receptor, and the ligand-activated receptor binds to DNA-response elements, which induce transcription (transactivation) of genes in all target cells. Most studies in clinical pharmacology of glucocorticoids attempt to develop compounds demonstrating good anti-inflammatory actions but low side effects. Changes in the molecular structure leading to an improvement in the efficacy mostly imply also higher side effect. As typical compounds, betamethasone dipropionate and clobetasol propionate may be mentioned. By increasing the lipid solubility by esterification, novel steroids such as budesonide, mometasone furoate, prednicarbat, 17,21-hydrocortisone aceponate and hydrocortisone-17-butyrate 21-propionate, methylprednisolone aceponate, alclometasone dipropionate, and fluticasone propionate have been developed with lower side effects (Brazzini and Pimpinelli 2002).

Some of the transcribed proteins after receptor binding, however, exert an indirect negative regulation of gene expression (transrepression) by activation of pro-inflammatory transcription factors that inhibit the anti-inflammatory activity of glucocorticoids (Schäcke et al. 2004). This effect offers the possibility to develop compounds with different activities in anti-inflammatory action and undesirable effects in future.

Cutaneous Manifestations. Under normal conditions, up to 99% of the applied topical glucocorticoid is removed form the skin by rubbing, washing off, and exfoliation, and only 1% is therapeutically active. Cutaneous adverse effects are always more pronounced in the face than in other areas of the body, since they increase the degradation of collagen and elastic fibres induced by sunlight. The aging skin is at higher risk than young skin. The following undesirable effects occur with different severity: skin atrophy and striae distensae, delayed wound healing, steroid acne and perioral dermatitis, erythema and teleangiectasias with petechia and ekchymosis, hypertrichosis, striae distensae, thinning of the skin, teleangiectasias, and – in the face – a rosacealike dermatitis. Tables 5.2 and 5.3 list summaries of adverse effects of topical steroids that are reported in the literature.

Atrophy, the most common adverse effect on the skin, appears as increased transparency, shininess of the skin, and the appearance of striae. The intensity of atrophy depends on age, body site, potency of topical glucocorticoids, and the presence of

Table 5.2 Adverse effects of topical glucocorticoids (Hengge et al. 2006)

Skin atrophy
Telangiectasia
Striae
Purpura
Stellate pseudoscars
Ulceration
Easy bruising
Masked microbial infections (tinea incognito)
Aggravation of cutaneous candidiasis, herpes, or demodex
Reactivation of Kaposi sarcoma
Granuloma gluteale infantum
Ocular hypertension
Glaucoma, cataract
Steroid rebound, steroid addiction, tachyphylaxis
Steroid acne
Perioral dermatitis
Steroid rosacea
Hirsutism
Hyperpigmentation
Hypopigmentation
Photosensitization
Rebound flare (psoriasis)

occlusion during steroid administration (Fig. 5.5). As a consequence, the skin surface becomes flat, and the rete ridges become straightened (Coßmann 2005; Fig. 5.6 a,b). The teleangiectasia and easy bruising is a direct consequence of the atrophy of the dermal tissue. In the oral cavity, angina bullosa haemorrhagica (oral blood blister) has been reported (Hanania et al. 1995). Subcutaneous injection of glucocorticoids may induce localized dents (Fig. 5.7).

The thinning of the horny layer barrier results in increased permeability, which accounts for an increased transepidermal water loss and a decreased synthesis of epidermal lipids. The thinning of the dermis may be up to 15% already after a few weeks of administration of potent glucocorticoids.

Hypertrichosis is rare, but variable degrees have been observed. Hypopigmentation is more significant in patients with dark skin; the lesions are generally reversible.

Disturbed wound healing by glucocorticoids is mainly due to the prevention of the early inflammatory phase, which is essential for efficient wound repair. The application of

Table 5.3 Reported adverse events of glucocorticoids in paediatric patients, according to an FDA report (Hengge et al. 2006)

Event in 202 patients	Frequency
Local irritation	66
Skin depigmentation or discoloration	30
Striae or skin atrophy	30
Cushing syndrome	6
Growth retardation	5
Hyperglycemia (diabetes)	5
Scarring	5
Staphylococcal infection	5
Genital hypertrichosis	4
Hirsutism	4
Rosacea	4
Acne	3
Glaucoma	3
Hypersensitivity reaction	3
Adrenal insufficiency	2
Bruising	2
Fungal infection	2
Gynecomastia	2
Perioral dermatitis	2
Mental status or mood change	2

glucocorticoids prior to wounding results in markedly decreased infiltration and activation of inflammatory cells.

As glucocorticoid therapy suppresses inflammation, fungal or bacterial growth flourishes. Also, worsening of herpes simplex, molluscum contagiosum, and scabies infection has been reported (Hengge et al. 2006). As a particular side effect of inhaled glucocorticoids, oropharyngeal candidosis may develop (Hanania et al. 1995).

Also, steroid acne, resulting from the degradation of the follicular epithelium and extrusion of the follicular contents, is common in glucocorticoid treatment, but it does not occur in Cushing syndrome. It is more frequently observed in younger patients and also after topical treatment. The acneiform eruption can be discriminated from the acne vulgaris by the lack of comedos (Feingold and Elias 1988; Hengge et al. 2006).

Perioral dermatitis is frequently found after abuse of topical glucocorticoids on the face (Fig. 5.8). Erythema and teleangiectasia together with the atrophy are usually seen only after topical use of glucocorticoids on the face over long periods. The manifestation begins with intermittent papules and pustules that are initially controlled with steroids of low potency. Subsequently, the lesions may prompt the continued use of steroids with

5

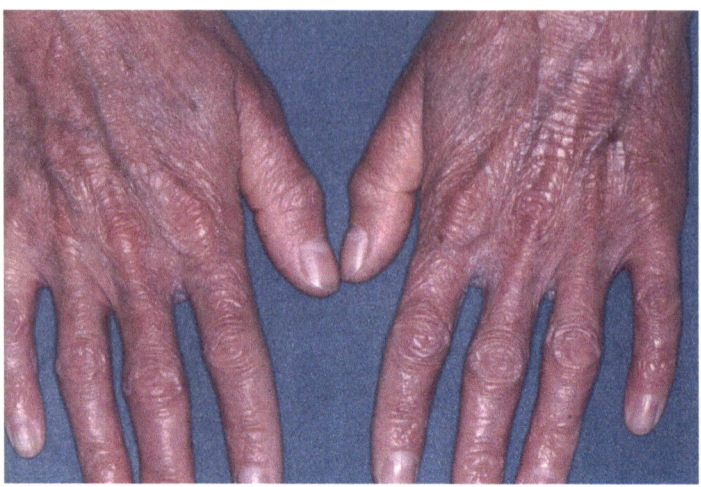

Fig. 5.5 Drug-induced hypercortisolism. Atrophy is the most common adverse effect on the skin. It appears as increased transparency, shininess of the skin, and the appearance of striae. The intensity of atrophy depends on age, body site, and potency of topical steroids

greater potency. The continued use of steroids may develop into a 'corticosteroid addiction'. Similarly, perioral dermatitis may develop, which is most frequently observed in young women.

Skin atrophy (but not striae), hypertrichosis, steroid acne, and rosacealike dermatitis are usually reversible after cessation of glucocorticoid treatment.

As a rare adverse effect, contact sensitization to topical glucocorticoids occurs. It was found in 2% (57/2838) of patients undergoing patch test because of allergic dermatitis. Ninety-three percent (53/57) of the patients reacted to a glucosteroid mixture, and four of them were positive only to individual glucocorticoids. The most common allergen was budesonide (Rocha et al. 2002). It seems that non-fluorinated glucocorticoids bear a higher risk of contact allergy than fluorinated compounds. Binding to the amino acid arginine as part of certain proteins seems to be a pre-requisite for allergic reactions to glucocorticoids. In the case of contact sensitization to topical glucocorticoid formulations, the hypersensitivity to other constituents, e.g. lanolin, preservatives, and antibiotics, has to be ruled out (Hengge et al. 2006).

Fear of adverse effects culminating in glucocorticoid phobia is not infrequent. Charman et al. (2000) studied the prevalence and source of phobia against topical glucocorticoids in 200 patients with atopic ekzema. The study comprised a questionnaire with three questions: (1) 'Do you worry about using steroid creams and ointments on your/your child's skin?' (2) 'If the answer is yes, why do you worry?' (3) 'Have your worries about steroid creams ever stopped you from using steroids prescribed by a doctor?' Question 1 was positively answered by 145 of 200 patients, and Question 3 by 48 of 145 patients. As an

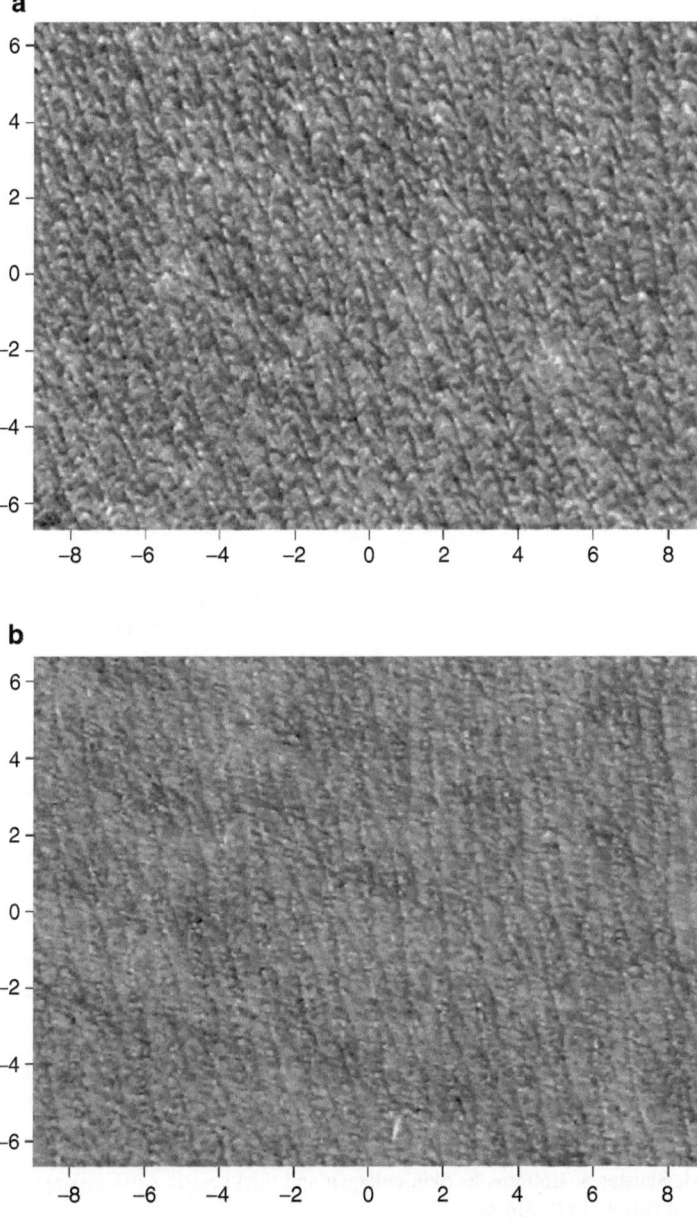

Fig. 5.6 Drug-induced hypercortisolism, topical glucocorticoid-induced atrophy. The skin surface becomes flat and the rete ridges become straightened. (**a**) Profile of skin surface, volar part of the arm, prior to treatment with clobetasol; (**b**) Profile of skin surface of the same area, after 4 weeks of treatment with clobetasol propionate. The roughness of the surface is significantly reduced (from Coßmann 2005, with permission)

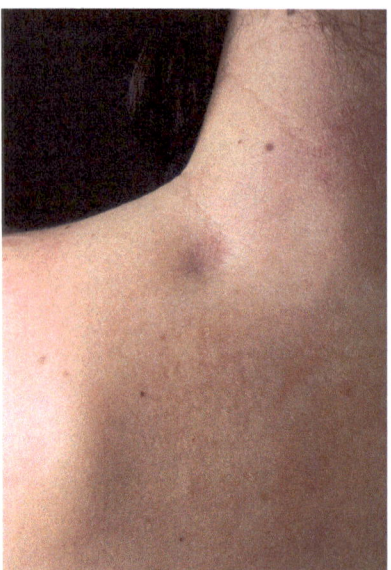

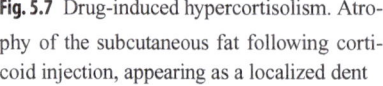

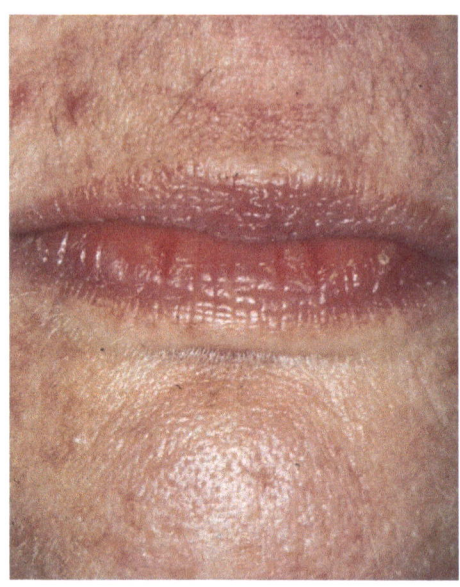

Fig. 5.7 Drug-induced hypercortisolism. Atrophy of the subcutaneous fat following corticoid injection, appearing as a localized dent

Fig. 5.8 Drug-induced hypercortisolism. Perioral dermatitis is frequently found after long-term application of topical glucocorticoids on the face

answer to Question 2, skin thinning was indicated by 34.5% and by unknown long-term effects in 24% of patients. In a second part of the questionnaire, a list of 12 commonly steroid formulations was presented and patients were asked to indicate which preparations they were currently using. The study does not provide information on the association of the steroids used and the worries, nor does it provide information of the patients' personal experience with adverse effects.

Treatment. The adverse effects of glucocorticoid treatment resolve spontaneously when the therapy ends. Additional treatment is not necessary.

References

Black MM, Shuster S, Bottoms E. Skin collagen and thickness in Cushing's syndrome. Arch Dermatol Forsch. 1973;246(4):365–8.

Brazzini B, Pimpinelli N. New and established topical corticosteroids in dermatology: clinical pharmacology and therapeutic use. Am J Clin Dermatol. 2002;3(1):47–58.

Burke WA, Briggaman RA, Gammon WR. Epidermolysis bullosa acquisita in a patient with multiple endocrinopathies syndrome. Arch Dermatol. 1986;122(2):187–9.

Charman CR, Morris AD, Williams HC. Topical corticosteroid phobia in patients with atopic eczema. Br J Dermatol. 2000;142(5):931–6.

Coßmann M. Messung von Hautatrophie unter vierwöchiger topischer Anwendung verschiedener Glukokortikosteroide mit Optischer Kohärenztomographie, Ultraschall und Profilometrie. Inauguraldissertation Lübeck 2005

Feingold KR, Elias PM. Endocrine-skin interactions. Cutaneous manifestations of adrenal disease, pheochromocytomas, carcinoid syndrome, sex hormone excess and deficiency, polyglandular autoimmune syndromes, multiple endocrine neoplasia syndromes, and other miscellaneous disorders. J Am Acad Dermatol. 1988;19(1 Pt 1):1–20.

Groves RW, MacDonald LM, MacDonald DM. Profound digital collagen atrophy: a new cutaneous presentation of adrenal-dependent Cushing's syndrome. Br J Dermatol. 1990;123(5):667–71.

Hanania NA, Chapman KR, Kesten S. Adverse effects of inhaled corticosteroids. Am J Med. 1995;98(2):196–208.

Hengge UR, Ruzicka T, Schwartz RA, Cork MJ. Adverse effects of topical glucocorticosteroids. J Am Acad Dermatol. 2006;54(1):1–15.

Jabbour SA. Cutaneous manifestations of endocrine disorders: a guide for dermatologists. Am J Clin Dermatol. 2003;4(5):315–31.

Kendereski A, Micic D, Sumarac M, Zoric S, Macut D, Colic M, Skaro-Milic A, Bogdanovic Z. White Addison's disease: what is the possible cause? J Endocrinol Invest. 1999;22(5):395–400.

Rocha N, Silva E, Horta M, Massa A. Contact allergy to topical corticosteroids 1995–2001. Contact Dermatitis. 2002;47(6):362–3.

Schäcke H, Docke WD, Asadullah K. Mechanisms involved in the side effects of glucocorticoids. Pharmacol Ther. 2002;96(1):23–43.

Schäcke H, Schottelius A, Docke WD, Strehlke P, Jaroch S, Schmees N, Rehwinkel H, Hennekes H, Asadullah K. Dissociation of transactivation from transrepression by a selective glucocorticoid receptor agonist leads to separation of therapeutic effects from side effects. Proc Natl Acad Sci U S A. 2004;101(1):227–32.

Shah SS, Oh CH, Coffin SE, Yan AC. Addisonian pigmentation of the oral mucosa. Cutis. 2005;76(2):97–9.

Sheu HM, Yu HS, Chang CH. Mast cell degranulation and elastolysis in the early stage of striae distensae. J Cutan Pathol 1991;18(6):410–6.

Shibli-Rahhal A, Van Beek M, Schlechte JA. Cushing's syndrome. Clin Dermatol. 2006;24(4):260–5.

Stratakis CA, Mastorakos G, Mitsiades NS, Mitsiades CS, Chrousos GP. Skin manifestations of Cushing disease in children and adolescents before and after the resolution of hypercortisolemia. Pediatr Dermatol. 1998;15(4):253–8.

Sunkel S, Wichmann-Hesse A, Gartner R, Hesse G. Pigmentvermehrung bei Schmidt-Syndrom (polyglanduläres Autoimmunsyndrom Typ II). Hautarzt. 2001;52(10 Pt 2):974–6.

Watson RE, Parry EJ, Humphries JD, Jones CJ, Polson DW, Kielty CM, Griffiths CE. Fibrillin microfibrils are reduced in skin exhibiting striae distensae. Br J Dermatol 1998;138(6):931–7.

Endocrine Hypertension, Pheochromocytoma

6

Synopsis

› Specific skin lesions were described in singular reports,
  e. g., multiple cutaneous metastases in malignant pheochromocytoma. An association with dermatomyositis, with Behcet syndrome, Sweet's syndrome, and erythema nodosum was reported.
› Pheochromocytoma is a frequent tumor in neurofibromatosis (NF) type 1 (see Sect. 14.4), described in 0.1–5.7% of the patients.

Aetiopathogenesis. Pheochromocytoma is not regularly associated with cutaneous symptoms. Specific effects of the enhanced levels of catecholamines have not been identified so far.

Pheochromocytoma is a frequent tumor in neurofibromatosis (NF) type 1 (see Sect. 14.4) that was described in 0.1–5.7% of patients. Patients with NF-associated pheochromocytomas are predominantly women in their early forties. While most patients have symptoms, 20% are asymptomatic. Although the majority of NF-associated pheochromocytomas are benign, approximately 11% are malignant, with metastasis at initial presentation. Thus, patients who present with episodes of hypertension, sweating, headache, and palpitation after diagnosis of NF1 should be evaluated for pheochromocytoma (Erem et al. 2007; Lew et al. 2006).

Cutaneous Manifestations. Specific skin lesions were described in singular reports. In a case of malignant pheochromocytoma, multiple cutaneous metastases were seen (Duquia et al. 2006).

A patient with skin manifestations resembling Addison's disease was observed by Zawar and Walvekar (2004). A 25-year-old man presented with skin pigmentation, which darkened on sun exposure. Additionally, he experienced intermittent episodes of excessive sweating, tremors, fatigue, and headache. On presentation, the skin showed slate-grey

Walter K. H. Krause, *Cutaneous Manifestations of Endocrine Diseases*,
DOI: 10.1007/978-3-540-88367-8, © Springer-Verlag Berlin Heidelberg 2009

macular pigmentation on the forehead, cheeks, nose, lips, helices, and dorsum of the hands. Scars of acne and previous injuries over the legs were also hyperpigmented. Further diagnostic efforts revealed an adrenal pheochromocytoma, which was surgically removed. The pigmentation faded rapidly in the immediate postoperative period, and the scar at the operation site did not pigment significantly. The authors speculated that pigmentation is a consequence of stimulation of melanocytes by a product of the pheochromocytoma, but they provided no details on the possible mechanism.

Naeyaert et al. (1987) reported on a patient with pheochromocytoma who was treated with the β-adrenoreceptor antagonist atenolol. He developed acral skin lesions; histologically, the lesions turned out as epidermal and sweat-gland necrosis, which resembled changes found in patients with carbon monoxide poisoning. They appeared to be the consequence of a combination of local ischemia and profuse sweating.

An association of dermatomyositis (Fig. 6.1), which, in general, is frequently associated with a malignant tumor in 3–60% of cases in different series, was reported by Yeh et al. (2001). Only 4 months after diagnosis, a malignant pheochromocytoma of the right adrenal gland was diagnosed. Kulp-Shorten et al. (1990) observed a case of leukocytoclastic vasculitis associated with multiple endocrine neoplasia type II. The lesions healed after removal of bilateral pheochromocytomas.

Random associations with pheochromocytoma may underlie the case reports in patients with Behcet's syndrome (Oishi et al. 1989; Bethea and Khan 1999), Sweet's syndrome (Fig. 6.2) (Dereure et al. 2004), and erythema nodosum (Gallego Dominguez et al. 2005).

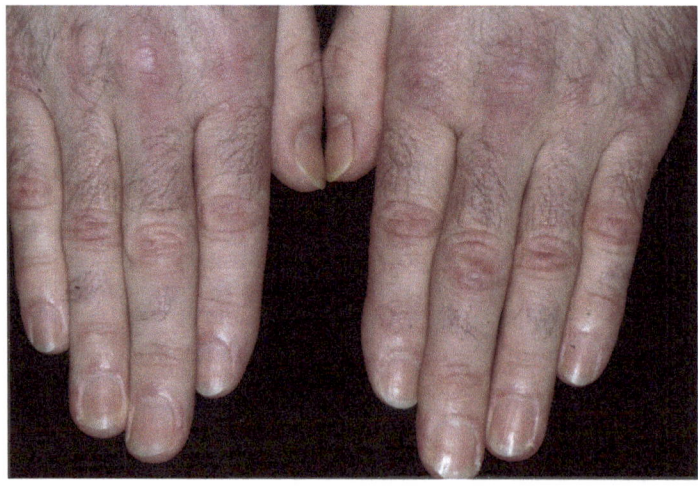

Fig. 6.1 Dermatomyositis in a patient with pheochromocytoma. There were flat, soft nodules of typical livid discoloration covering the joints of the fingers

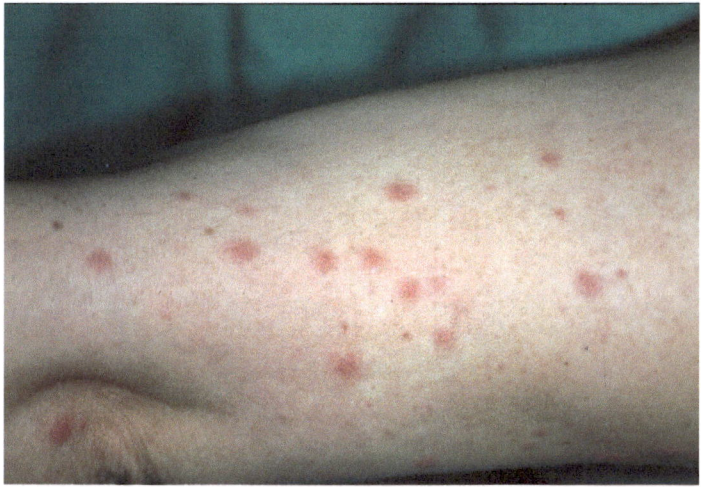

Fig. 6.2 Sweet's syndrome in a patient with pheochromocytoma. Subepidermal pustules are aggregated in red, flat plaques and nodules

References

Bethea L, Khan S. Behcet's disease and pheochromocytoma. J S C Med Assoc. 1999;95(8):295–8.

Dereure O, Ebrard-Charra S, Guillon F, Baldet P, Guilhou JJ. Sweet's syndrome associated with pheochromocytoma. Dermatology. 2004;208(2):175.

Duquia RP, de Almeida HL Jr, Traesel M, Jannke HA. Cutaneous metastasis of pheochromocytoma in multiple endocrine neoplasia IIB. J Am Acad Dermatol. 2006;55(2):341–4.

Erem C, Onder Ersoz H, Ukinc K, Hacihasanoglu A, Alhan E, Cobanoglu U, Kocak M, Erdol H. Neurofibromatosis type 1 associated with pheochromocytoma: a case report and a review of the literature. J Endocrinol Invest. 2007;30(1):59–64. Review.

Gallego Dominguez S, Pascua Molina FJ, Caro Mancilla A, Gonzalez Nunez A. Erythema nodosum becoming a pheochromocytoma. Ann Med Int. 2005;22(8):383–6.

Kulp-Shorten CL, Rhodes RH, Peterson H, Callen JP. Cutaneous vasculitis associated with pheochromocytoma. Arthritis Rheum. 1990;33(12):1852–6.

Lew JI, Jacome FJ, Solorzano CC. Neurofibromatosis-associated pheochromocytoma. J Am Coll Surg. 2006;202(3):550–1.

Naeyaert JM, Derom E, Santosa S, Rubens R. Sweat-gland necrosis after beta-adrenergic antagonist treatment in a patient with pheochromocytoma. Br J Dermatol. 1987;117(3):371–6.

Oishi S, Koga B, Sasaki M, Umeda T, Sato T. Pheochromocytoma associated with Behcet's disease. Jpn J Clin Oncol. 1989;19(3):283–6.

Yeh CN, Jeng LB, Chen MF, Hung CF. Nonfunctioning malignant pheochromocytoma associated with dermatomyositis: case report and literature review. World J Urol. 2001;19(2):148–50.

Zawar VP, Walvekar R. A pheochromocytoma presenting as generalized pigmentation. Int J Dermatol. 2004;43(2):140–2.

Androgens

7

Synopsis

Androgens in the Male

> Hypogonadism causes delay of puberty and reduced growth and/or function of genital organs, terminal hairs, male voice, and male sexuality. Substitution of testosterone induces pubertal development, growth of target organs, and gain of function similar to the normal course.

> In age-related androgen deficiency (age-related hypogonadism), the texture of the skin becomes smooth and fine wrinkles occur. The terminal hairs are not reduced, but the sebaceous glands show markedly reduced function. A testosterone supplementation is justified only when hypogonadal symptoms are verified by low testosterone levels. It should be performed with percutaneous substitution.

> Androgenetic alopecia, the loss of scalp hairs, is a very common disease, beginning typically with bitemporal recession, followed by progressive thinning in the frontal and vertex areas of the scalp (male pattern baldness). It is triggered by high local levels of dihydrotestosterone. The inhibition of dihydrotestosterone synthesis by finasteride is effective in preventing further hair loss during the early stages of baldness, and re-growth also has been observed.

> Acne fulminans is clearly associated with hyperandrogenism. It is characterized by inflammatory nodules and plaques that undergo rapid suppuration, together with acute illness, fever, and musculoskeletal manifestations. Systemic glucocorticoids have been most effective therapy together with antibiotics. Isotretinoin is of little use in acne fulminans.

Androgen Excess in the Female

> Androgen excess is one of the most frequent problems in women of reproductive age, affecting approximately 7% of the population. The most frequent causative disease in about 80% of these cases is polycystic ovary syndrome (PCOS).

Continued

Walter K. H. Krause, *Cutaneous Manifestations of Endocrine Diseases*,
DOI: 10.1007/978-3-540-88367-8, © Springer-Verlag Berlin Heidelberg 2009

7

> Seborrhoea is very common. The diagnosis is based mainly on the clinical impression; a measurement of the amount of sebum covering the skin surface is not performed in clinical practice. Antiandrogen treatment lowers total skin surface lipids.

> Acne, occurring predominantly on the face and on the neck, back, and chest, is due to enhanced androgenic stimulation of the sebaceous glands. Elevated androgen levels have been reported in 30% to 90% of females with acne. Oral contraceptives are recommended as treatment. Ethinyl estradiol has been used as an estrogen in most studies; the most effective progestin is cyproterone acetate (not available in the United States).

> Hirsutism in women is defined as an increase in facial and body hair that exceeds an aesthetically acceptable level. It is a clinical marker of enhanced androgen production. In idiopathic hirsutism, ovulatory function and circulating androgen concentrations are normal. Various endocrine regimens have been described as treatment.

> Female pattern hair loss (androgenetic alopecia) is not always associated with androgen excess. It is characterized by diffuse thinning in the frontal and parietal areas of the scalp and by a central pattern of scalp hair loss; however, in contrast to male pattern alopecia, the frontal area is usually preserved. Topical application of estrogens may be useful as treatment. The 5 -reductase inhibitor finasteride is ineffective.

Dehydroepiandrosterone

> Dehydroepiandrosterone (DHEA) and its sulphate ester DHEA-S are hormonal inactive precursors of steroid hormones.

> Direct effects to the skin are questionable, and only minor effects were demonstrated in cell culture. Serum levels of DHEA-S are 100 to 500 times higher than those of testosterone, and decrease continuously with aging. This observation provoked the interest in supplementation of DHEA in aging men and women.

> Although some effects were described in uncontrolled observations, the benefits observed were scarce in placebo-controlled studies. Reliable effects were found in the treatment of systemic lupus erythematosus.

7.1
Androgens in the Male

7.1.1
Hypogonadism

Aetiopathogenesis. Hypogonadism designates reduced growth and function of genital organs. The most important causes are:

(1) Idiopathic hypogonadotropic hypogonadism (IHH), based on impairment of secretion of GnRH from the hypothalamus. As a consequence, the gonadotropin secretion from the pituitary fails and, secondarily, the testicular testosterone production is insufficiently activated. The incidence is approximately 1 in 10^6 boys. A considerable number of syndromes (OMIM gives 62 hits) is known, in which skin changes are associated with hypogonadism and possibly additional endocrinopathies. The most relevant of these will be outlined in Chap. 14.
(2) Klinefelter syndrome, induced by one or more supernumerary X-chromosomes. The most frequent karyotype is 47,XXY or a mosaic 47,XXY/46,XY (Velissariou et al. 2006). It is the most frequent numeral chromosome abnormality, with an incidence of 1 in 500 boys. The patients are generally infertile.
(3) Androgen receptor defects.

The consequence of the abnormalities is reduced or absent stimulation of the target organs for testosterone, i.e. genital organs, terminal hairs, larynx, and muscles. The clinical consequences are delay of puberty, and a lack of growth of genital organs and development of functions, terminal hairs, male voice, and male sexuality.

Cutaneous Manifestations. Boys with IHH do not undergo pubertal changes. The growth of the genital organs, the pubic and axillary hairs, body hairs, and the beard does not start within the age of 12 to 14 years, when normal puberty takes place. These boys do not develop acne and pubertal gynecomastia. Untreated older patients do not develop androgenetic alopecia. The middle phalanges remain hairless. These features are also seen, to various degrees, in patients with androgen receptor defects (Köhn et al. 2000).

Patients with Klinefelter syndrome usually develop normal pubertal signs. Signs of androgen deficiency occur similar to that in androgen deficiency of the aging male (see below), but in earlier years of life. As a special feature, they have a higher risk of the development of leg ulcers (Downham and Mitek 1986; Veraart et al. 1994). Klinefelter syndrome is also a risk factor for male breast cancer. The prevalence of male breast cancer is approximately 50 times higher than in normal males (Hultborn et al. 1997).

Treatment. The substitution of testosterone in hypogonadism induces pubertal development similar to the normal course. The patients evolve all signs of adult males, including genital growth, growth of pubic and axillary hairs, body hairs, the beard, and prevalence of acne. The administration of GnRH in a pulsatile fashion, or of gonadotropins, is also able to overcome all the dysfunctions, including infertility.

In Klinefelter syndrome, testosterone substitution is advisable in earlier years rather than in the aging male. Leg ulcers in Klinefelter syndrome are treated as leg ulcers in general. Guidelines for chronic wounds have to be considered.

In the case of androgen receptor defects, no treatment is possible so far (Holterhus et al. 2000).

7.1.2
Androgen Deficiency of the Aging Male

Aetiopathogenesis. The Massachusetts Male Aging Study (MMAS) demonstrated that testosterone levels decline with aging, at a range of about 1% per year in the age span from 40 to 70 years of life. The decline is steeper in men with chronic illness and otherwise compromised health. As a counterpart, the levels of SHBG increase (McKinlay et al. 1989). The mechanisms and clinical implications of this phenomenon are still under debate; it is still unclear whether a syndrome of hypogonadism of the aging male (late-onset hypogonadism) exists. A complete cessation of androgen secretion occurs as a consequence of orchidectomy or drug-induced androgen deprivation for treatment of androgen-dependent prostate cancer.

Cutaneous Manifestations. The age-related androgen deficiency in the male rarely causes skin manifestations. The beard hairs do not decrease in the skin area covered and in the speed of renewal, although the interval between shaving usually increases (Fig. 7.1). The axillary hairs and the sebaceous glands, however, show markedly reduced function; as a paradox, the hyperplastic sebaceous glands increase. The texture of the skin becomes smooth, and fine wrinkles occur (Fig. 7.2). Complete cessation of testicular androgen secretion may also induce hot flushes similar to those observed after female menopause.

Treatment. Low testosterone production in the aging male requires testosterone supplementation. A treatment is justified only when hypogonadal symptoms occur in combination with low testosterone levels. In recent years, it is well accepted that testosterone supplementation should be performed with percutaneous substitution. Several different testosterone gel formulations are available in the market. The amount applied should be varied in accordance to the testosterone serum levels; as an average dose, the application

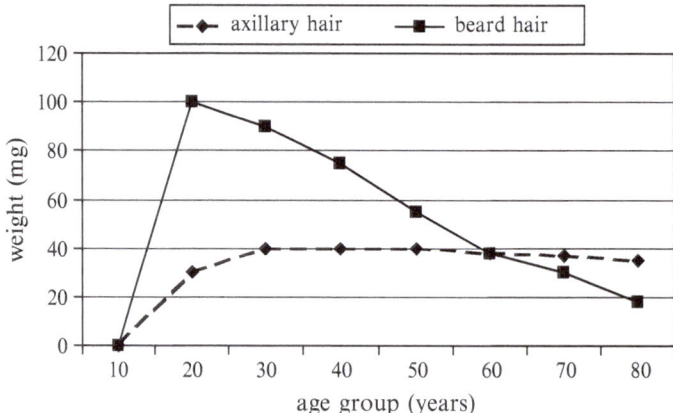

Fig. 7.1 Different patterns of androgen-dependent hair growth in the beard and the axilla. While beard growth continues at high levels into old age, axillary hair growth is maximal in the mid-twenties, and decreases slowly with aging (depicted from Randall 2007)

Fig. 7.2 In male aging, in parallel to the decrease of testosterone levels, the texture of the skin becomes smooth, and fine wrinkles occur

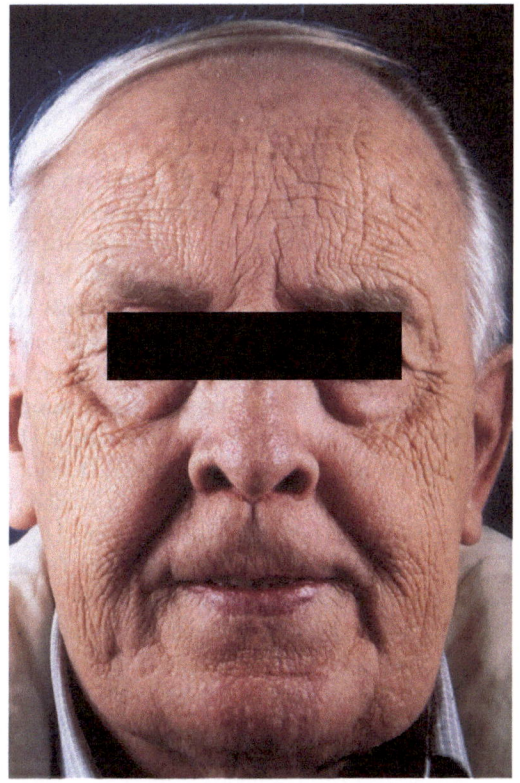

of 5 g gel containing 5 mg of testosterone is recommended (Nieschlag et al. 2005). Effects of testosterone substitution on skin changes are not yet described. The hot flushes improve with treatment with cyproterone acetate, which is already used as a therapeutic tool in androgen deprivation (Feingold and Elias 1988).

7.1.2.1
Androgenetic Alopecia

Aetiopathogenesis. Androgenetic alopecia (AGA) describes the loss of hairs from androgen-sensitive hair follicles.

Hair follicles undergo a growth cycle through various stages of proliferation (anagen), involution (catagen), and resting (telogen). In the anagen phase, the hair shaft is growing, and most epithelial compartments of the hair follicle undergo proliferation. During the catagen stage, the hair follicles undergo controlled involution, characterized by apoptosis of epithelial cells and condensation of the dermal papilla. In the telogen phase, the hair shaft changes to a club hair, which is mostly shed from the follicle. After this, the growth cycle starts again. AGA is characterized by progressive shortening of the duration of anagen with successive hair cycles, leading to decreased numbers of hair in anagen at any given time, and progressive follicular miniaturization with conversion of terminal to vellus-like follicles (Hoffmann, 2002; Trüeb 2002).

In a normal adult scalp, the anagen phase lasts from 2 to as long as 7 years. In men with AGA, the duration of anagen decreases from several years to months or weeks, while the telogen phase remains of the same duration. This leads to a marked reduction in the anagen-to-telogen ratio, from a normal 6 to 8:1 ratio to an abnormal 0.1 to 3:1 ratio. Moreover, the lag period between the telogen and anagen phase becomes progressively longer, leading to a reduction in the number of hairs present on the scalp at any one time (Kaufman 2002).

More than 50 years ago, Hamilton concluded that hair growth in some regions of the scalp is androgen-dependent, based on his observation that castrated men did not develop AGA, but that this manifestation appeared if the castrated men were treated with testosterone. The hair follicles and the sebaceous glands, together designated as a pilosebaceous unit, are the most important androgen-sensitive structure of the skin. Hair follicles have 3 types of androgen-dependency: (1) androgen-insensitive follicles on the eyelashes and hair of the occipital head; (2) androgen-dependent hair follicles that grow on androgenic stimulation, e. g. beard or axillary hairs; (3) androgen-sensitive hair follicles, in which the anagen phase is shortened by androgens; the terminal hair regresses to vellus hair, e. g. hair of the frontal scalp (Hoffman 2004). In addition, the androgen-dependent hair follicles require different levels of testosterone, e. g. axillary hairs are sufficiently stimulated by only low levels in the female range, while beard hairs require higher levels in the male. The individual androgen-sensitivity of follicles also changes. In boys and hirsute women, the initial alteration of facial follicles concerns those above the mouth and on the chin; eventually, the alteration spreads over the lower face and parts of the neck. Many androgen responses are gradual, with some follicles taking years to manifest full response (Randall 2007).

The phenomenon that androgens stimulate hair follicles in many areas, but has no effect in others, and inhibits the same organ in another part of the body, is yet poorly explainable. It may be due to different genetic sensitivity, and may result from a combination of elements that determine different responsiveness of hair follicles to androgen. The dermal papilla, derived from the mesenchym, appears to play a central role in determining the androgen-sensitivity of hair follicles from different sites (Alonso and Rosenfield 2003; Zouboulis and Degitz 2004; Randall 2007).

Dihydrotestosterone plays a key role in the pathogenesis of male androgenetic alopecia. The 5α-reductase irreversibly converts testosterone to 5α-dihydrotestosterone. Two isoforms of the enzyme have been described. In hair follicles, the membrane-bound 5α-reductase type 2, encoded by the *SRD5A2* gene located at band p23 on chromosome 2, is active. Men with testosterone deficiency and men with genetic 5α-reductase deficiency do not develop androgenetic alopecia (Kaufman 2002). The identical enzyme is also active in the prostate gland; thus, an association of the risk of both prostate diseases and male pattern baldness exists. Chen et al. (2004) investigated 46 patients, aged 56–87 years, and benign prostatic hyperplasia (BPH) was diagnosed on grounds of an enlarged prostatic volume (>30 ml) and decreased maximal urine flow rate (< 15 mg/s). These patients had a higher prevalence of androgenetic alopecia than a control group with small prostates. A correlation of prostate size to the degree of androgenetic alopecia did not exist. This observation, however, does not imply a general association of the two diseases. Hayes et al. (2007) observed a polymorphism of the gene (A49T) that was associated with a greater risk of prostate cancer than the was wild type, but a lower risk of androgenetic alopecia (Hamilton–Norwood scale). Another polymorphism (V89L) was associated with neither an enhanced risk of prostate cancer nor of alopecia.

Androgen metabolism is only one of the pathogenic factors of AGA. Several recent studies underlined the implication of microscopic follicular inflammation in the pathogenesis of AGA. These processes may lead to irreversible damage to the follicular stem cells in the 'bulge' area of the outer root sheath in the superficial portion of the hair follicle. AGA also has genetic implications, but the genetic mechanisms and predisposition remain poorly understood. It is also unclear whether AGA is genetically homogeneous (Trüeb 2002). Table 7.1 schematically summarizes the etiopathogenetic factors of AGA.

Cutaneous Manifestation. Male pattern baldness is a very common disease. For clinical purposes, stages are distinguished according to the Norwood–Hamilton scale (www. keratin.com). Male pattern hair loss typically begins with bitemporal recession, preceding to a recession of the frontal border of hair, followed by progressive thinning in the frontal and vertex areas of the scalp (Fig. 7.3). Over time, the frontal and vertex thinning areas may merge, resulting in near-complete visible hair loss over the top of the scalp (Kaufman 2002).

Histopathology. The histopathological characteristics of AGA include an increase in follicular stelae, increased numbers of vellus, and reduced numbers of terminal hairs, but signs of inflammation and scarring are scarce (Fig. 7.4). The first phase of miniaturization of terminal hairs is frequently associated with perifollicular lymphocytic infiltration, and possibly fibrosis (Tosti et al. 1999; Trüeb 2002).

Treatment. Effective pharmacological treatment of AGA is possible with two drugs: minoxidil and finasteride. The two drugs do not cure AGA, but medical treatment with finasteride or minoxidil should be continued indefinitely. The vertex of the scalp is the area that is most likely to respond to treatment, with little or no hair regrowth occurring on the anterior scalp or at the hairline.

During treatment of hypertension with minoxidil, hypertrichosis was noted as a side effect. This observation encouraged dermatologists to develop a topical formulation that was purported to arrest progression of the hair loss and regrow hair in approximately 90% of men. The large placebo effects, however, cast doubt on these results, and may be explained by insufficient techniques to evaluate hair growth. Much of the regrowth was of cosmetically insignificant indeterminate hairs, but progression of the balding was stopped. Treatment must be maintained for at least 6 months before any assessment of efficacy. When the patient ceases treatment, all these new hairs are shed. The combination of topical

Table 7.1 Etiopathogenic factors of AGA (Trüeb 2002)

Genetic factors	Polygenic transmission, androgen receptor formation, steroidogenic enzymes
Environmental factors	androgens, microbes, irritants, UV irradiation (?)
Dermal papilla	fibroblasts, follicular epithelium, cytokines, stem cell apoptosis, perifollicular fibrosis

7

Fig. 7.3 Androgenetic alopecia
(AGA). In the male, the hair loss
comprises the occipital region and
frontal receding hairline
("Geheimratsecken")

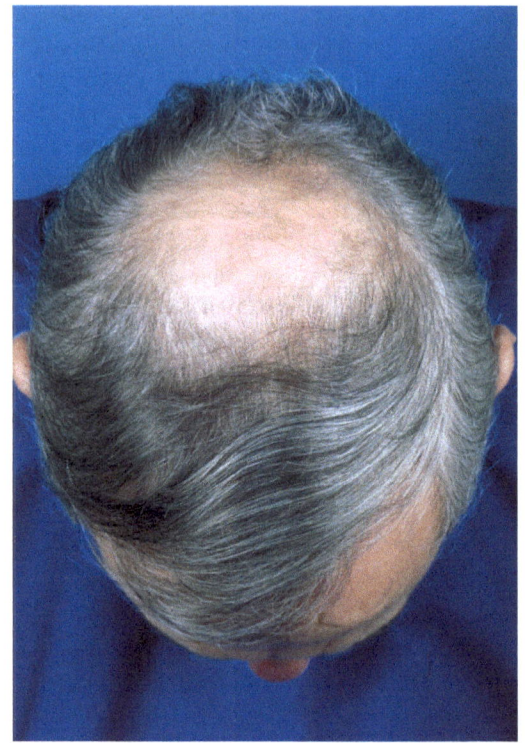

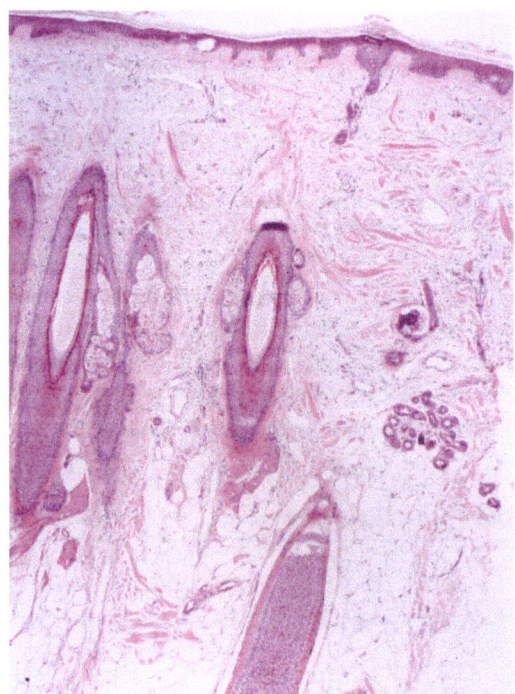

Fig. 7.4 Androgenetic alopecia
(AGA). Histopathology showed
increased number of vellus hairs
in the scalp skin

minoxidil with topical tretinoin is limited by irritation of the scalp, and the benefits have not been substantiated in large studies. Topical minoxidil has few side effects; only skin irritation and, rarely, contact allergic dermatitis have been observed (Sinclair 1998; Scow et al. 1999; Tosti et al. 1999).

Finasteride, which inhibits the conversion of testosterone to dihydrotestosterone, was introduced for the treatment of prostatic hyperplasia. As it is active in much the same manner in the scalp skin (Drake et al. 1999), it was also applied for the treatment of AGA. In studies, finasteride was effective in preventing further hair loss during the early stages of baldness, but regrowth was also observed in 24-month trials. Sexual side effects (decreased libido and erectile dysfunction) were indicated by 3.8% of patients treated, compared to 2.1% of the placebo group (Scow et al. 1999; Tosti et al. 1999; Hoffmann and Happle 2000).

It remains to be clarified whether the use of finasteride for AGA in the third and forth decade of life will influence prostate growth and the incidence of BPH, as a mean decrease of PSA serum levels by 50% and in men aged 44–57 years by 50% was observed in the verum group, but no decrease in the placebo group (D'Amico and Roehrborn 2007). Chen et al. (2004) hypothesized that the long-term use of finasteride for AGA might lower the incidence of BPH in these patients.

In severe AGA, full head or partial hairpieces, real or synthetic hair, as well as different techniques of surgical transplantation of follicles from skin with androgen insensitive hairs (Tosti et al. 1999) are options.

7.1.3
Acne Fulminans

Aetiopathogenesis. Acne is not possible without androgens. Androgens active in the skin are derived from dehydroepiandrosterone sulphate (DHEA-S) and androstenedione, which are predominantly produced in the adrenal glands, and from testosterone, which is mainly synthesized in the gonads. In the skin, a steroid sulphatase metabolizes DHEA-S to DHEA. Subsequently, 3β-hydroxysteroid dehydrogenase/D5/4-isomerase 3 converts DHEA to androstenedione. A 17-βhydroxysteroid dehydrogenase then metabolizes androstenedione testosterone. Finally, 3α-hydroxysteroid-dehydrogenase, an enzyme existing in three isoforms, catabolizes active androgens to compounds that do not bind to the androgen receptor. The presence of androgen receptors was demonstrated in epidermal and follicular keratinocytes, sebocytes of the sebaceous glands, sweat gland cells, dermal papilla cells, dermal fibroblasts, endothelial cells of the vascular structures, and genital melanocytes (Zouboulis and Degitz 2004).

Juvenile acne, which occurs in 90% of all boys, relies also on other factors, such as increased sebum production, abnormal follicular epithelial differentiation, and cornification obstructing the pilosebaceous follicle by desquamated epithelial cells. Subsequently, the follicular microorganisms (e.g., *Propionibacterium acnes*) flourish, and inflammation follows as the follicle ruptures and sebum products attain the dermis.

The severity of acne is not correlated to circulating testosterone serum levels. However, over-dosage of exogenous androgens increases the occurrence of acne. The abuse of anabolic-androgenic steroids (AAS) in bodybuilders, who administrate the drugs with the aim of enhancing muscle mass, induces more severe features of acne. More than 50% of users exhibit acne papulopustulosa, acne conglobata, or acne fulminans. Each appearance of severe acne in young men should be taken as a possible hint of AAS use (Melnik et al. 2007). Also, the administration of androgens as a treatment for excessive height in boys, which produced testosterone serum levels of two or three times above the normal range, induced acne in 64% of the boys (Traupe et al. 1988; Hartmann and Burg 1989).

In particular, acne fulminans is clearly associated with hyperandrogenism. In addition, special immune defects and associations with HLA antigens have been discussed in the literature (Davis et al. 1981; Piazza and Giunta 1991; Wong et al. 1992). Some authors have suggested that acne fulminans represents an abnormal immunologic response to acnes. Testosterone administration raised the size of sebaceous glands and thus induced an increase in the population density of propionibacterium acnes (Heydenreich 1989). AAS-induced acne may be worsened by oral or parenteral administration of vitamin preparations containing high doses of vitamin B2, B6, and B12.

Cutaneous Manifestations. Acne fulminans is characterized by acute illness, fever, and musculoskeletal manifestations. It presents with acute onset of inflammatory nodules and plaques, lesions undergo rapid suppuration, leaving ragged hemorrhagic ulcers, which leave large atrophic scars at the site of ulcerative lesions (Fig. 7.5). Typically, it affects

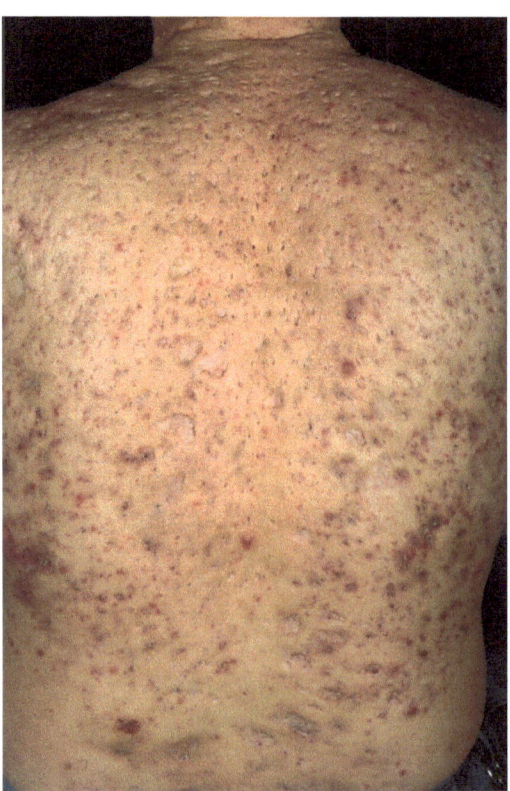

Fig. 7.5 Acne fulminans. Scars following the massive inflammatory, abscess-like lesions with ulcers and crusts

male adolescents with a history of mild to moderate acne. Patients frequently have general symptoms such as fever, malaise, arthralgias, and myalgias. Aseptic, osteomyelitis-like, osteolytic bone lesions have also been reported in these patients (Mehrany et al. 2005). It is different from acne conglobata, and occurs almost exclusively in boys.

Treatment. Systemic glucocorticoids are the most effective therapy to control the cutaneous, constitutional, and musculoskeletal symptoms (Pinzer and Hahn 1983; Mehrany et al. 2005), together with antibiotics such as clindamycin, erythromycin, and tetracycline. Diclofenac was also of benefit (Piazza and Giunta 1991). Interestingly, isotretinoin is of little use in acne fulminans, and even deterioration of the diseases with the use of isotretinoin has been described (Heydenreich 1989). The clearance of the lesions in the skin and in the musculoskeletal system usually takes several months.

7.2
Androgen Excess in the Female

Incidence of Androgen Excess. Androgen excess is one of the most frequent problems in women of reproductive age, affecting approximately 7% of the population. In 873 patients who claimed to suffer from clinical features of androgen excess, polycystic ovary syndrome (PCOS) was the most frequent causative diseases in 82% of the women. Of these patients, 22.2% had no endocrine abnormalities, while increased testosterone or DHEA-S levels were found in the remaining. A reliable association of clinical features to different endocrine values (levels of total testosterone, free testosterone, DHEA-S) was not found (Azziz et al. 2004). Carmina et al. (2006) reported on 950 unselected women with clinical signs of androgen excess at two endocrine departments. Of these patients, 72.1% were diagnosed as having PCOS, 15.8% as having idiopathic hyperandrogenism, 7.6% as having idiopathic hirsutism, 4.3% as having 21-hydroxylase-deficient nonclassic adrenal hyperplasia, and 0.2% (1 case) as having androgen-secreting tumours.

The incidences of the clinical features of androgen excess as outlined below are different. The prevalence of acne in women declines with age, from approximately 90% of women at age 18 years of age to 10% of women at 45 years of age. Female pattern hair loss affects approximately 5% of women by the age of 50, and the rate increases to more than 30% by the age of 70.

7.2.1
Seborrhoea

Aetiopathogenesis. Seborrhoea, resulting from enhanced activity of the sebaceous glands due to androgenic stimulation, is very common (Fig. 7.6). It is rarely recognized as a disease per se by patients and physicians, but it is usually observed in combination with acne. In principle, the skin surface lipids originate from two sources: the secretion of the sebaceous glands, the sebum, and the lipids of the keratinocytes. The precise physiologic function of sebum is not known. The epidermal lipids are important for the intercellular cohesion of corneocytes, and thus are responsible for the water-proofing of the cutis.

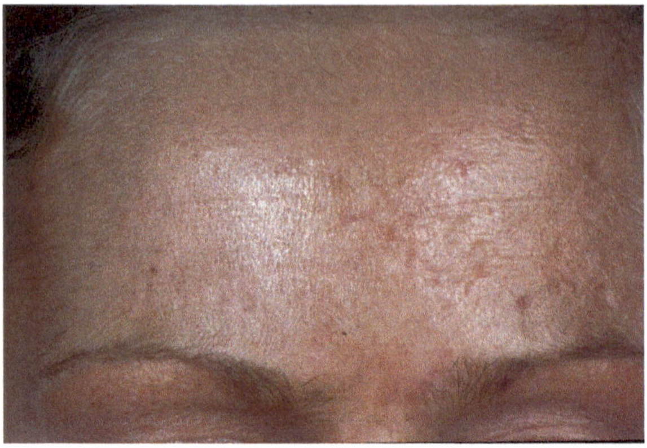

Fig. 7.6 Seborrhea. The skin is shining, fatty, and covered with an oil-like sebum. The diagnosis is based mainly on the clinical impression; a measurement of the amount of sebum covering the skin surface is not performed in clinical practice

Cutaneous Manifestation. The diagnosis of seborrhoea is based mainly on the clinical impression; a measurement of the amount of sebum covering the skin surface is not performed in clinical practice. Determination of the amount and analysis of the composition of skin surface lipids is possible after extraction by organic solvents from the skin surface, absorption to films, and photometric methods, which are based on the increased transparency of frosted glass or a plastic sheet after application of lipids to the surface (Clarys and Barel 1995; Piérard et al. 2000).

Treatment. Antiandrogen treatment lowers total skin surface lipids (Patel and Noble 1987). A specific treatment of seborrhoea per se is not necessary.

7.2.2
Acne

Aetiopathogenesis. Elevated androgen levels have been reported in 30% to 90% of females with acne. Acne in patients below the age of 20 is more likely to be due to androgenic excess. (Slayden et al. 2001). The authors studied 30 consecutive unselected postmenarchal women with acne (without hirsutism) and 24 eumenorrhoeic healthy controls that were age-matched. There was no significant correlation between the severity of acne and age, BMI, or hormonal values. Patients had significant lower median levels of SHBG and higher median levels of free T and DHEA-S than controls. There was no difference in the median total testosterone levels between acne patients and controls. Overall, 19 patients had at least one elevated androgen. Similar to these findings, other investigators have reported high levels of free testosterone and high levels of DHEA-S in patients with acne without hirsutism, but few other studies have reported the presence of essentially normal androgen levels in acne patients without hirsutism (Slayden et al. 2001).

Like in boys (see Chap.7), juvenile acne is not an endocrine disease in girls, but it also relies on other factors such as increased sebum production, abnormal follicular epithelial differentiation, cornification obstructing the pilosebaceous follicle by desquamated epithelial cells, and the augmentation of follicular microorganisms (e.g., *Propionibacterium acnes*).

Cutaneous Manifestation. Acne occurs predominantly on the face and, to a lesser extent, on the neck, back, and chest (Fig. 7.7). The clinical feature as well as treatment possibilities will not be described here in detail, but the reader is referred to textbooks on dermatology.

Treatment. Endocrine therapeutic regimens act via depression of androgen production or androgen effects on the sebaceous glands (Thielitz and Gollnick 2005). Haider and Shaw (2004) reviewed controlled studies on the effectiveness of estrogen–gestagen combinations, as used in oral contraceptives, for treating acne. They were able to decrease inflammatory lesions by approximately 50%, or even more, after a treatment period of 6 months. Ethinyl estradiol was chosen as the estrogen in most studies, while various progestins such as cyproterone acetate, drospirenone, levonorgestrel, drospirenone, and desogestrel were used. Oral contraceptives containing chlormadinone have been shown to be superior to oral contraceptives containing levonorgestrel in treating acne. The safety profile of all combination drugs is good. Cardiovascular risks are not significantly increased in nonsmokers, and breast cancer risks have not been shown to be increased, overall. However, there is an increased risk of deep vein thrombosis.

Beneficial effects on acne have been documented with the antiandrogen cyproterone acetate (which is not available in the United States), buserelin, flutamid, and spironolactone (Poulin, 2004). The success rate was similar to that obtained with oral contraceptives. For further treatment modalities of acne, the reader is referred to textbooks on dermatology.

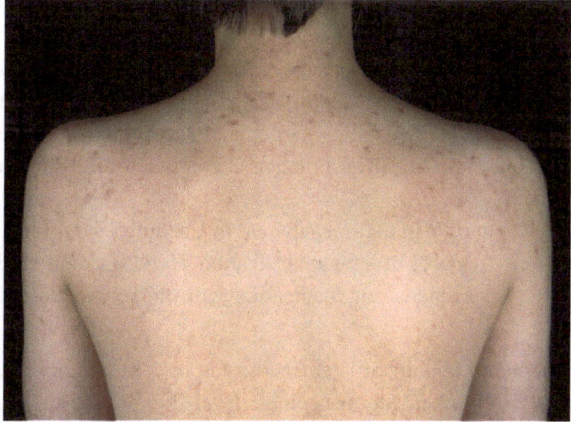

Fig. 7.7 Acne. Inflammatory papules with abscess formation strictly linked to the pilosebaceous units

7.2.3
Hirsutism

Aetiopathogenesis. The most frequent cause of hirsutism is PCOS. Souter et al. (2004) measured total and free testosterone, dehydroepiandrosterone sulphate, 17-hydroxy-progesterone, sex hormone-binding globulin, and basal insulin and glucose levels in 228 women with minimal unwanted hair growth. Of the patients, 54% demonstrated a disease indicating androgen excess; in 50% of the cases, this was polycystic ovary syndrome. It is concluded that an endocrine evaluation is also justified in women with minimal unwanted hair growth. In the study of Taponen et al. (2003), 10.4% of women reporting hirsutism had biochemical abnormalities. The subjects who reported both oligomenorrhoea and hirsutism (3.4%) had the highest testosterone, LH, and insulin levels, the highest free androgen index, and the lowest SHBG levels. In a study of 100 women aged 18–50 years (Birch et al. 2006), 30 subjects had no hair problems, 41 had typical female pattern hair loss alone, and 29 had facial hirsutism. Of the hirsute women, 13 also had scalp hair loss. Hirsute women had significantly higher androgen levels than non-hirsute women. In non-hirsute women, there was no difference in androgen levels between those with and without scalp hair loss. The BMI was elevated in hirsute women, compared with non-hirsute women. There was no significant difference in sebum excretion between women without hirsutism and hirsute women with normal androgen levels. There was no correlation between hair density and sebum excretion.

Hirsutism is suggested to be a clinical marker of enhanced androgen production, but the correlation is not very close (Azziz et al. 2004). Approximately half of mild hirsutism and most moderately severe hirsutism cases are associated with increased serum androgen levels. As the response of the pilosebaceous unit to androgen varies individually, some women with moderately elevated levels of androgen have no skin manifestation of androgen excess, while others have acne or alopecia. On the other hand, idiopathic hirsutism may be associated with normal androgen levels, if the hair follicle is more sensitive to androgen (Alonso and Rosenfield 2003).

Idiopathic hirsutism is defined as hirsutism with normal ovulatory function and normal circulating androgen concentrations. A history of regular menses is not sufficient; ovulatory function must be confirmed by using a daily basal body temperature charting and/or a luteal phase (day 20–24 of the menstrual cycle) progesterone level (Azziz et al. 2000). Approximately 15% to 30% of hirsute women do not have ovulatory abnormalities, and usually have normal levels of circulating androgens. These women are generally considered to have idiopathic hirsutism (The Practice Committee of the American Society for Reproductive Medicine 2004).

Hirsutism may also appear in acromegaly and in Cushing's syndrome. Hirsutism may be combined with other features of female virilization. Hypertrichosis similar to hirsutism may also occur as a consequence of medication with minoxidil, diazoxide, phenytoin, cyclosporine, and danazol.

Cutaneous Manifestation. Hirsutism is defined as an increase in facial and body hair in women that exceeds an aesthetically acceptable level (Fig. 7.8). This applies only if the areas involved are identical to the male androgen-dependent hairs (beard, upper trunk, lower abdomen, thighs). Other forms of hypertrichosis that do not appear in androgen-sensitive

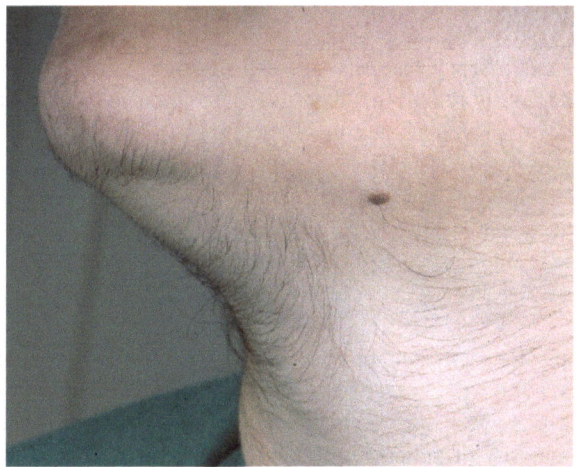

Fig. 7.8 Hirsutism. An increase in facial and body hair in women in the areas of androgen-dependent hairs (beard, upper trunk, lower abdomen, thighs) that exceeds an aesthetically acceptable level

areas have to be separated. The definition depends on the ethnic background. It is a weak definition, given that as many as one third of women complain of excess facial hair. After menopause, the incidence increases further ("witch hairs") (Feingold and Elias 1988).

A quantification of hirsutism is possible with the score described by Ferriman and Gallwey (1961). The density of terminal hairs at 11 different body sites (upper lip, chin, chest, upper back, lower back, upper abdomen, lower abdomen, arm, forearm, thigh, and lower leg) is estimated. In each of these areas, a score of 0 (absence of terminal hairs) through 4 (extensive terminal hair growth) is assigned. Later studies deleted the areas of the forearm and lower leg. Scoring of hair growth in the sideburn area, lower jaw, upper neck, and buttocks have been included in more recent scoring systems. From these data, a sum score of 8 or more has been considered to represent hirsutism (Azziz et al. 2000). In a study including 369 patients, 7.6%, 4.6%, and 1.9% demonstrated a modified Ferriman–Gallwey score of >6, 8, or 10, respectively. Hirsutism in Asian women is relatively uncommon, even when similar metabolic and endocrine abnormalities are present. In these women, the absence of hirsutism cannot be used to exclude the presence of a hyperandrogenic disorder.

Treatment. Endocrine treatment of hirsutism follows several lines.

- For hormonal abnormalities, a correction of abnormal hormone production is desirable.
- Estrogen–progestin preparations as used in oral contraceptives are recommended as a first-line therapy by the Practice Committee of the American Society for Reproductive Medicine (2004). Cyproterone acetate as an antiandrogen may be administered only in combination with ethinyl estradiol as an oral contraceptive. Finasteride is precluded, because of its significant teratogenic potential.

- Long-acting GnRH agonists suppress the hypothalamic-pituitary-ovarian axis in severely androgenized patients. This expensive treatment is restricted to rare patients. The therapy is usually combined with estrogen–progestin oral contraceptives.
- Corticosteroid suppression is useful in patients with adrenocortical hyperactivity (persistently elevated levels of DHEA-S).
- Insulin-sensitizing agents are indicated in patients with additional insulin resistance, which is frequent in patients with PCOS.
- Ketoconazole is able to suppress ovarian and adrenal androgen biosynthesis, but it also suppresses the secretion of other adrenal hormones.

Hormonal therapy alone will sometimes produce a thinning and a loss of pigmentation of terminal hairs, but it will generally not cause terminal hairs to revert to vellus hairs. Approximately 80% to 90% of patients will note a cessation in the progression of their hirsutism. The majority of patients will also observe variable degrees of slowing in the rate of hair growth. The treatment success is reversible when hormonal treatment is stopped.

Approximately 20% of patients with androgen excess do not respond to the initial hormonal therapy within 6 to 8 months of beginning treatment. In these patients and also in those with idiopathic hirsutism, topical treatments that modulate hair growth may be applied. There are number of methods, summarized in Table 7.2.

Eflornithine, the first substance applicable for topical modulation of unwanted hair growth, was originally synthesized as an anti-cancer drug, and was later used in the African disease, sleeping sickness. Hair loss was observed as a side effect in the treated patients. Eflornithine inhibits the ornithin decarboxylase, resulting in a reduction of the length of the anagen phase (Jobanputra et al. 2007). Eflornithine is applied topically as a 13.9% cream. It is frequently used in combination with laser treatment, and randomized comparative studies clearly showed the superiority of the combination to the laser treatment without eflornithine (Smith et al. 2006; Hamzavi et al. 2007). As side effects, mild local reactions, but no generalized adverse effects, were observed (Wolf et al. 2007).

Table 7.2 Topical methods of reduction of unwanted hair growth (from Kunte and Wolff 2001)

Mechanical: Waxing, epilation razoring, abrasion
Chemical: Thioglycolate, bleaching
Electrical: Electrolysis, thermolysis
Laser photothermolysis: Alexandrite laser, Neodym-YAG laser, Ruby laser, Diode laser
Pulsed light: Flashlamps
Drugs: Eflornithin

7.2.4
Androgenetic Alopecia

Aetiopathogenesis. Female pattern hair loss (FPHL) is generally thought to be the female equivalent of male balding, and is often termed androgenetic alopecia. Although hair loss is common in hyperandrogenetic women, it is questionable whether FPHL is associated in all cases with other clinical or biochemical signs of androgen excess (Birch et al. 2006). Genetic determinants seem to predominate.

Hair loss may be associated with other cutaneous signs of androgen excess, including hirsutism and acne, in only a minority of women. These women may benefit from antiandrogen therapy. In a study of 873 hyperandrogenic women, only 4% had scalp hair loss, whereas hirsutism was present in 75% (Birch et al. 2006). Women with typical FPHL, however, do not generally present with other clinical symptoms of hyperandrogenism, and serum testosterone levels are usually within the normal range. Also, a 1-year, placebo-controlled study with finasteride in postmenopausal women with FPHL demonstrated no clinical benefit on scalp hair growth, compared to treatment with placebo. This observation underlines that hair loss is less closely associated to hyperandrogenism than hirsutism.

Cutaneous Manifestation. FPHL, presenting usually in the later decades of life, is characterized by diffuse thinning in the frontal and parietal areas of the scalp and by a central pattern of scalp hair loss; however, in contrast to male pattern alopecia, the frontal area is usually preserved (Fig. 7.9). Complete baldness is rarely observed in premenopausal women with FPHL. Postmenopausal women may develop a pattern more similar to male pattern hair loss (Kaufman 2002).

Treatment. The topical application of estrogens may be useful, but do not effectively prevent or control androgenetic alopecia in women. Only a few controlled studies are available. Local side effects are rare; pruritus is sometimes observed. The effect is due to the induction of the aromatase in the hair follicles, which causes an increased metabolism of testosterone to estradiol (Alonso and Rosenfield 2003).

The 5α-reductase inhibitor finasteride, which is effective in the treatment of male balding, was less effective only in a small case series of hyperandrogenic women with female pattern hair loss. In a large controlled trial in postmenopausal women with normal androgen levels, finasteride failed to halt the progression of hair loss. Also, cyproterone acetate was not superior to placebo in a controlled study (Birch et al. 2006).

7.3
Dehydroepiandrosterone

Aetiopathogenesis. Dehydroepiandrosterone (DHEA) and its sulphate ester DHEA-S are hormonal inactive precursors of steroid hormones, which are secreted in large amounts from the adrenal glands. They may be converted into potent androgens and/or estrogens in peripheral tissues. In fact, plasma DHEA-S levels in adult men and women are 100–500 times higher than those of testosterone and 1,000–10,000 times higher than those of estradiol, thus providing a large reservoir of substrate. Serum levels of DHEA and DHEA-S decrease

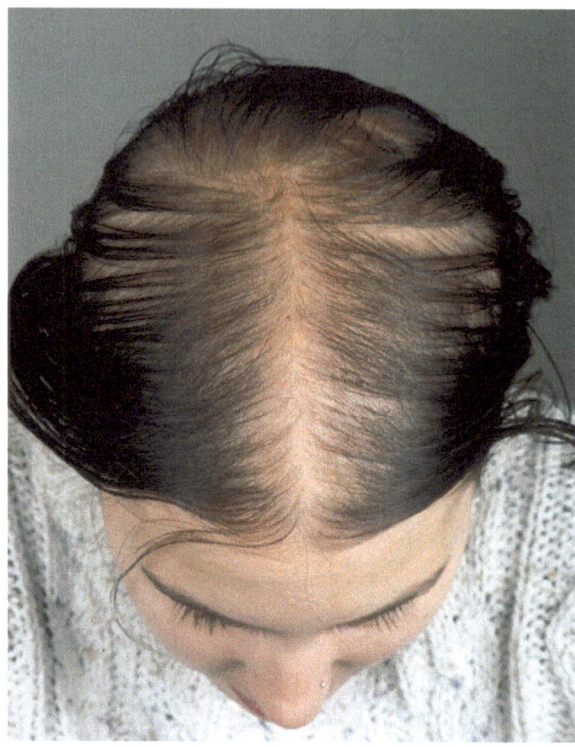

Fig. 7.9 Androgenetic alopecia. Female pattern alopecia is characterized by diffuse thinning of the hairs in the frontal and parietal areas of the scalp

continuously with aging, suggesting an association between skin aging and DHEA levels (Labrie et al. 2005).

Some in vitro studies attempted to find evidence for a direct effect of DHEA on skin cells. By experimental treatment of human dermal fibroblasts with 10 mM DHEA for 24, 48, and 72 h, the expression of type I procollagen and tissue inhibitor of matrix metalloprotease protein (TIMP-1) were increased, and matrix metalloproteinases protein MMP-1 was decreased. While UV irradiation decreased type I procollagen expression and induced the expression of MMP-1 protein in culture, DHEA treatment (50 mM) significantly prevented the downregulation of type I procollagen and also inhibited UV induction of MMP-1 protein expression on the mRNA level (Lee et al. 2000; Shin et al. 2005). In vivo, the topical application of DHEA also increased the expressions of type I procollagen mRNA and protein in human skin. Topical DHEA treatment significantly reduced MMP-1 mRNA expression. In vivo, DHEA also increased the expressions of TGF-β1 and the connective tissue growth factor (CTGF) mRNA in cultured human dermal fibroblasts and human skin.

Shin et al. (2005) summarized the results of their study in connection with others:

(1) DHEA stimulates procollagen and TIMP-1 protein production and decreases MMP-1 expression in cultured fibroblasts.
(2) DHEA prevents UV-induced changes of MMP-1 and procollagen expression by inhibiting UV-induced AP-1 activation.
(3) The topical application of DHEA in aged human skin increases procollagen and TIMP-1 levels and reduces MMP-1 expression.
(4) Topical application of DHEA increases TGF-β1 and CTGF expression to induce procollagen synthesis in aged skin.

Consequently, the authors are strongly convinced that DHEA is a candidate agent for the prevention and treatment of clinical changes in intrinsic aging and photoaging, such as skin wrinkles and skin laxity.

Results of Supplementation. DHEA has been shown to have important effects on the skin of aged individuals. Topical treatment with DHEA cream for 12 months in 15 women between the ages of 60 to 70 years led to a slight increase in skin thickness by 10%, and sebum secretion increased by 73%. Systemic effects on body weight, muscle mass, and lipoproteins were not observed.

Sebum production increases also following systemical DHEA supplementation. The index of sebum secretion was 79% higher after 12 months of DHEA therapy, with a return to pre-treatment values 3 months after cessation of treatment. This has been shown in a number of studies performed in women, particularly those over 70 years old who are physiologically hyposeborrhoeic. The DHEA-induced increase in sebum production is probably because the sebaceous glands contain all the steroidogenic enzymes necessary to catalyze the conversion of DHEA to testosterone and dihydrotestosterone. Other beneficial effects of DHEA supplementation on the skin have been noticed: skin hydration increased, while skin dryness (which makes the skin rough) and skin pigmentation decreased (Labrie et al. 2005). The oral administration of DHEA for a year improved skin status in the elderly, particularly in woman, in terms of hydration, epidermal thickness, sebum production, and pigmentation (Shin et al. 2005).

It remains unclear whether beneficial effects are due to DHEA directly, or whether they occur only after metabolization to testosterone and estrogens. Labrie et al. (2005) formulated that "the advantage of treating skin changes with DHEA is the fact that the compound it metabolized to androgen or estrogen only in the hormone-dependent tissues that possess the metabolizing enzymes".

The largest randomized study on DHEA treatment was published by Baulieu et al. (2000). In this double-blind study, 280 healthy individuals of both genders, aged 60–79 years, were given DHEA 50 mg daily, or given a placebo for a year. Skin parameters were measured parallel to blood and urine samples, immune parameters, biomarkers for bone metabolism, (IGF-1), homocysteine, cholesterol, HDL-cholesterol, triglycerides, glycaemia, creatininaemia, hepatic function, and other hormones at different times. Table 7.3 shows that statistically significant superiority of DHEA treatment over placebo administration was demonstrated in sebum production, skin hydration, and skin pigmentation, but only in women over 70 years old.

Table 7.3 Effects of DHEA supplementation for a year on three cutaneous parameters in the DHEAge study (Baulileu et al. 2000)

	Placebo	DHEA	Probability of significance
All volunteers			
Sebum production, no. of spots	61 (11.7–132)	101 (44.2–161.5)	0.0008
Skin hydration (forearm)	71 (70.7–89.8)	86 (74.5–96)	0.01
Skin pigmentation (face)	15.9 (14.8–17.4)	15.3 (14.2–16.6)	0.02
Men < 70 years			
Sebum production, no. spots	114 (67–157)	155 (97–177)	0.11
Skin hydration (forearm)	77.5 (69–88.5)	86.5 (78–98)	0.03
Skin pigmentation (face)	16 (4.2–16.8)	15 (14–16.5)	0.26
Men > 70 years			
Sebum production, no. spots	132.7 (65–172)	109 (75–172)	0.64
Skin hydration (forearm)	87 (73.4–100)	87 (77.5–96.5)	0.58
Skin pigmentation (face)	15.3 (14.8–16.5)	15.5 (14.3–16.7)	0.58
Women < 70 years			
Sebum production, no. spots	24.7 (10.9–65.4)	70.8 (21.7–162)	0.007
Skin hydration (forearm)	80 (71.5–85.7)	77.6 (71.7–94.9)	0.44
Skin pigmentation (face)	15.9 (14.4–17.2)	16 (15–17.1)	0.85
Women > 70 years			
Sebum production, no. spots	8.7 (1.8–47.2)	52.4 (26–105)	0.0001
Skin hydration (forearm)	78.3 (69.7–89.9)	85.7 (76.5–102.6)	0.07
Skin pigmentation (face)	16.9 (15.3–17.7)	15.1 (14.1–16)	0.003

Sebum was measured by using white adherent tape (Sebutape; CuDerm, Dallas), which is applied on defatted forehead skin. Absorbed lipids become visible as transparent spots, which are measured by using image analysis. Each spot corresponds to one active sebaceous gland. Skin surface hydration was evaluated by the measurement of electrical conductance of high-frequency electric current. Skin pigmentation (skin color) was determined by the technique of chromometry, according to a three-dimensional L, a*, b* reference CIE standard system.

DHEA is possibly active in the treatment of systemic lupus erythematosus (SLE, Fig. 7.10). The endocrine effects due to the peripheral conversion to androgenic and estrogenic sex steroids, and the immune modulating effects of DHEA by regulating the production of the Th-1 cytokines such as IL-2, both suggest that this hormone could be of benefit for patients with SLE. Several controlled studies and a number of observations have been published in this field. They equivocally suggested an effect on frequency of flares and on osteoporosis (induced by the glucocorticoids that were used for treatment). The useful dose added up to 200 mg/day for 7 to 12 months. There were side effects to the skin such as acne and hirsutism, but they were mild and well tolerated (van Vollenhoven 2002).

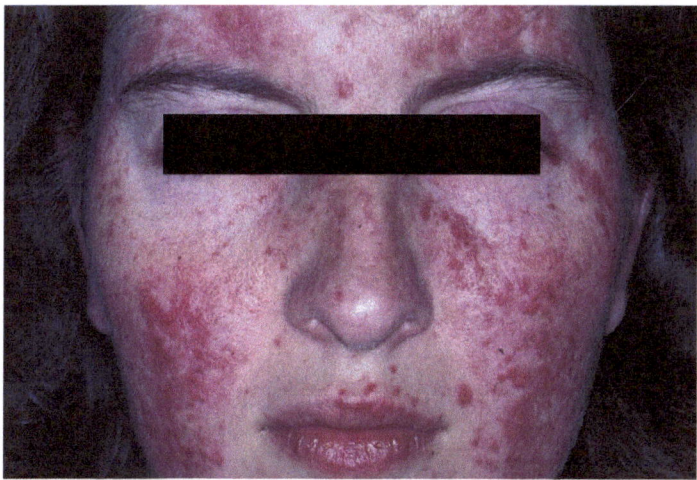

Fig. 7.10 Skin lesions of systemic lupus erythematosus (SLE). The lesions appear as soft, red patches with little scaling, predominantly in the light-exposed areas. They may change in size within a few days

References

Alonso LC, Rosenfield RL. Molecular genetic and endocrine mechanisms of hair growth. Horm Res. 2003;60(1):1–13.

Azziz R, Carmina E, Sawaya ME. Idiopathic hirsutism. Endocr Rev. 2000;21(4):347–62.

Azziz R, Sanchez LA, Knochenhauer ES, Moran C, Lazenby J, Stephens KC, Taylor K, Boots LR. Androgen excess in women: experience with over 1000 consecutive patients. J Clin Endocrinol Metab. 2004;89(2):453–62.

Baulieu EE, Thomas G, Legrain S, Lahlou N, Roger M, Debuire B, Faucounau V, Girard L, Hervy MP, Latour F, Leaud MC, Mokrane A, Pitti-Ferrandi H, Trivalle C, de Lacharriere O, Nouveau S, Rakoto-Arison B, Souberbielle JC, Raison J, Le Bouc Y, Raynaud A, Girerd X, Forette F. Dehydroepiandrosterone (DHEA), DHEA sulfate, and aging: contribution of the DHEAge Study to a sociobiomedical issue. Proc Natl Acad Sci U S A. 2000;97(8):4279–84.

Birch MP, Lashen H, Agarwal S, Messenger AG. Female pattern hair loss, sebum excretion and the end-organ response to androgens. Br J Dermatol. 2006;154(1):85–9.

Carmina E, Rosato F, Jannì A, Rizzo M, Longo RA. Extensive clinical experience: relative prevalence of different androgen excess disorders in 950 women referred because of clinical hyperandrogenism. J Clin Endocrinol Metab. 2006;91(1):2–6.

Chen W, Yang CC, Chen GY, Wu MC, Sheu HM, Tzai TS. Patients with a large prostate show a higher prevalence of androgenetic alopecia. Arch Dermatol Res. 2004;296(6):245–9.

Clarys P, Barel A. Quantitative evaluation of skin surface lipids. Clin Dermatol. 1995;13(4):307–21.

D'Amico AV, Roehrborn CG. Effect of 1 mg/day finasteride on concentrations of serum prostate-specific antigen in men with androgenic alopecia: a randomised controlled trial. Lancet Oncol. 2007;8(1):21–5.

Davis DE, Viozzi FJ, Miller OF, Blodgett RC. The musculoskeletal manifestations of acne fulminans. J Rheumatol. 1981;8(2):317–20.

Downham TF 2nd, Mitek FV. Chronic leg ulcers and Klinefelter's syndrome. Cutis. 1986;38(2):110–1.

Drake L, Hordinsky M, Fiedler V, Swinehart J, Unger WP, Cotterill PC, Thiboutot DM, Lowe N, Jacobson C, Whiting D, Stieglitz S, Kraus SJ, Griffin EI, Weiss D, Carrington P, Gencheff C, Cole GW, Pariser DM, Epstein ES, Tanaka W, Dallob A, Vandormael K, Geissler L, Waldstreicher J. The effects of finasteride on scalp skin and serum androgen levels in men with androgenetic alopecia. J Am Acad Dermatol. 1999;41(4):550–4.

Feingold KR, Elias PM. Endocrine-skin interactions. Cutaneous manifestations of adrenal disease, pheochromocytomas, carcinoid syndrome, sex hormone excess and deficiency, polyglandular autoimmune syndromes, multiple endocrine neoplasia syndromes, and other miscellaneous disorders. J Am Acad Dermatol. 1988;19(1 Pt 1):1–20.

Ferriman D, Gallwey JD Clinical assessment of body hair growth in women. J Clin Endocrinol Metab. 1961;21: 1440–7

Haider A, Shaw JC. Treatment of acne vulgaris. JAMA. 2004;292(6):726–35.

Hamzavi I, Tan E, Shapiro J, Lui H. A randomized bilateral vehicle-controlled study of eflornithine cream combined with laser treatment versus laser treatment alone for facial hirsutism in women. J Am Acad Dermatol. 2007;57(1):54–9.

Hartmann AA, Burg G. Acne fulminans bei Klinefelter-Syndrom unter Testosteron. Eine Nebenwirkung der Antihochwuchstherapie. Monatsschr Kinderheilkd. 1989;137(8):466–7.

Hayes VM, Severi G, Padilla EJ, Morris HA, Tilley WD, Southey MC, English DR, Sutherland RL, Hopper JL, Boyle P, Giles GG. 5-Alpha-reductase type 2 gene variant associations with prostate cancer risk, circulating hormone levels and androgenetic alopecia. Int J Cancer. 2007;120(4):776–80.

Heydenreich G. Testosterone and anabolic steroids and acne fulminans. Arch Dermatol. 1989;125(4):571–2.

Hoffmann R. Male androgenetic alopecia. Clin Exp Dermatol. 2002;27(5):373–82.

Hoffman R. Androgenetische Alopezie. Hautarzt. 2004;55(1):89–111

Hoffmann R, Happle R. Current understanding of androgenetic alopecia. Part I: etiopathogenesis. Eur J Dermatol. 2000;10(4):319–27.

Holterhus PM, Sinnecker GH, Hiort O. Phenotypic diversity and testosterone-induced normalization of mutant L712F androgen receptor function in a kindred with androgen insensitivity. J Clin Endocrinol Metab. 2000;85(9):3245–50.

Hultborn R, Hanson C, Köpf I, Verbiené I, Warnhammar E, Weimarck A. Prevalence of Klinefelter's syndrome in male breast cancer patients. Anticancer Res. 1997;17(6D):4293–7.

Jobanputra KS, Rajpal AV, Nagpur NG. Eflornithine. Indian J Dermatol Venereol Leprol. 2007;73(5):365–6.

Kaufman KD. Androgens and alopecia. Mol Cell Endocrinol. 2002;198(1–2):89–95.

Köhn FM, Ring J, Schill WB. Dermatologische Aspekte des Hypogonadismus. Hautarzt. 2000;51(4):223–30.

Kunte C, Wolff H. Aktuelle Therapie der Hypertrichosen. Hautarzt. 2001;52(11):993–7.

Labrie F, Luu-The V, Belanger A, Lin SX, Simard J, Pelletier G, Labrie C. Is dehydroepiandrosterone a hormone?. J Endocrinol. 2005;187(2):169–96.

Lee KS, Oh KY, Kim BC. Effects of dehydroepiandrosterone on collagen and collagenase gene expression by skin fibroblasts in culture. J Dermatol Sci. 2000;23(2):103–10.

McKinlay JB, Longcope C, Gray A. The questionable physiologic and epidemiologic basis for a male climacteric syndrome: preliminary results from the Massachusetts Male Aging Study. Maturitas. 1989;11(2):103–15

Mehrany K, Kist JM, Weenig RH, Witman PM. Acne fulminans. Int J Dermatol. 2005;44(2):132–3.

Melnik B, Jansen T, Grabbe S. Abuse of anabolic-androgenic steroids and bodybuilding acne: an underestimated health problem. J Dtsch Dermatol Ges. 2007;5(2):110–7.

Nieschlag E, Swerdloff R, Behre HM, Gooren LJ, Kaufman JM, Legros JJ, Lunenfeld B, Morley JE, Schulman C, Wang C, Weidner W, Wu FC. Investigation, treatment and monitoring of late-onset hypogonadism in males. Aging Male. 2005;8(2):56–8.

Patel S, Noble WC. Analysis of human skin surface lipid during treatment with anti-androgens. Br J Dermatol 1987;117:735–40.

Piazza I, Giunta G. Lytic bone lesions and polyarthritis associated with acne fulminans. Br J Rheumatol. 1991;30(5):387–9.

Piérard GE, Piérard-Franchimont C, Marks R, Paye M, Rogiers V. EEMCO guidance for the in vivo assessment of skin greasiness. The EEMCO Group. Skin Pharmacol Appl Skin Physiol. 2000;13(6):372–89.

Pinzer B, Hahn FS. Acne fulminans. Dermatol Monatsschr. 1983;169(2):136–8.

Poulin Y. Practical approach to the hormonal treatment of acne. J Cutan Med Surg. 2004;8 Suppl 4:16–21.

Randall VA. Hormonal regulation of hair follicles exhibits a biological paradox. Semin Cell Dev Biol. 2007;18(2):274–85.

Scow DT, Nolte RS, Shaughnessy AF. Medical treatments for balding in men. Am Fam Physician. 1999;59(8):2189–94, 2196.

Shin MH, Rhie GE, Park CH, Kim KH, Cho KH, Eun HC, Chung JH. Modulation of collagen metabolism by the topical application of dehydroepiandrosterone to human skin. J Invest Dermatol. 2005;124(2):315–23.

Sinclair R. Male pattern androgenetic alopecia. BMJ. 1998;317(7162):865–9.

Slayden SM, Moran C, Sams WM Jr, Boots LR, Azziz R. Hyperandrogenemia in patients presenting with acne. Fertil Steril. 2001;75(5):889–92.

Smith SR, Piacquadio DJ, Beger B, Littler C. Eflornithine cream combined with laser therapy in the management of unwanted facial hair growth in women: a randomized trial. Dermatol Surg. 2006;32(10):1237–43.

Souter I, Sanchez LA, Perez M, Bartolucci AA, Azziz R. The prevalence of androgen excess among patients with minimal unwanted hair growth. Am J Obstet Gynecol. 2004;191(6):1914–20.

Taponen S, Martikainen H, Jarvelin MR, Laitinen J, Pouta A, Hartikainen AL, Sovio U, McCarthy MI, Franks S, Ruokonen A. Hormonal profile of women with self-reported symptoms of oligomenorrhea and/or hirsutism: Northern Finland birth cohort 1966 study. J Clin Endocrinol Metab. 2003;88(1):141–7.

The Practice Committee of the American Society for Reproductive Medicine. The evaluation and treatment of androgen excess. Fertil Steril 2004;82(Suppl. 1):S173–80

Thielitz A, Gollnick H. Systemische Aknetherapie. Hautarzt. 2005;56(11):1040–7.

Tosti A, Camacho-Martinez F, Dawber R. Management of androgenetic alopecia. J Eur Acad Dermatol Venereol. 1999;12(3):205–14.

Traupe H, von Mühlendahl KE, Brämswig J, Happle R. Acne of the fulminans type following testosterone therapy in three excessively tall boys. Arch Dermatol. 1988;124(3):414–7.

Trüeb RM. Molecular mechanisms of androgenetic alopecia. Exp Gerontol. 2002;37(8–9):981–90

van Vollenhoven RF. Dehydroepiandrosterone for the treatment of systemic lupus erythematosus. Expert Opin Pharmacother. 2002;3(1):23–31.

Velissariou V, Christopoulou S, Karadimas C, Pihos I, Kanaka-Gantenbein C, Kapranos N, Kallipolitis G, Hatzaki A. Rare XXY/XX mosaicism in a phenotypic male with Klinefelter syndrome: case report. Eur J Med Genet. 2006;49(4):331–7.

Veraart JC, Hamulyak K, Neumann HA, Engelen J. Increased plasma activity of plasminogen activator inhibitor 1 (PAI-1) in two patients with Klinefelter's syndrome complicated by leg ulcers. Br J Dermatol. 1994;130(5):641–4.

7

Wolf JE Jr, Shander D, Huber F, Jackson J, Lin CS, Mathes BM, Schrode K; Eflornithine HCl Study Group. Randomized, double-blind clinical evaluation of the efficacy and safety of topical eflornithine HCl 13.9% cream in the treatment of women with facial hair. Int J Dermatol. 2007;46(1):94–8.

Wong SS, Pritchard MH, Holt PJ. Familial acne fulminans. Clin Exp Dermatol. 1992;17(5):351–3.

Zouboulis CC, Degitz K. Androgen action on human skin – from basic research to clinical significance. Exp Dermatol. 2004;13(Suppl 4):5–10.

Estrogens

8

Synopsis

Hyperestrogenism in the Male

> Hyperestrogenism in the male induces gynaecomastia, an enlargement of the male breast. It may be unilateral or bilateral. The term gynaecomastia is used for all types, irrespective of the consistence and the degree of swelling. It is important to differentiate benign gynaecomastia from male breast cancer. The treatment of choice is surgical removal of the enlarged tissue; pharmacological treatment gives no reliable results.

> As differential diagnoses, various diseases of the male nipple are mentioned, which are not related to hyperestrogenism.

Estrogens in the Female

> During the female climacteric, the skin becomes atrophic, and an average linear decline of collagen content of 2.1% per postmenopausal year has been described. Wrinkles, atrophy, laxity, and vulvar atrophy and dryness develop, due to reduction of the skin surface lipids. The changes can be revised with hormone replacement therapy (HRT), but topical administration may also exert beneficial effects to the skin. Phytoestrogens may confer positive estrogen-like effects, with fewer adverse effects.

> The existence of autoimmune estrogen dermatitis is not generally accepted. The proof that it is an autoimmune disease has not yet been met. The hallmark of the varying clinical picture is the cyclic premenstrual flare. Intradermal tests are necessary to establish the diagnosis. Treatment focuses on suppression of estrogen production.

> Unilateral nevoid teleangiectasia is a rare disease. It appears frequently in the last trimenon of pregnancy. Clinically, distributed singular teleangiectatic lesions in circumscribed areas, predominantly in the upper trunk and arms of only one side of the body, are observed. Treatment is possible with laser light.

Continued

Walter K. H. Krause, *Cutaneous Manifestations of Endocrine Diseases*,
DOI: 10.1007/978-3-540-88367-8, © Springer-Verlag Berlin Heidelberg 2009

> **Synopsis** *Continued*

> › Melanoma and estrogens: Estrogen receptors are present in melanoma, but melanoma is not an estrogen-dependent tumor. The determination of estrogen receptor status and a treatment with tamoxifen is not useful in the management of malignant melanomas. Melanoma cannot be regarded as a contraindication for HRT.

8.1
Hyperestrogenism in the Male

8.1.1
Gynaecomastia

Aetiopathogenesis. Gynaecomastia is an enlargement of the male breast. The term is derived from the Greek words "γψνε"(women) and "μαστοσ"(breast). The discrimination between gynaecomastia and lipomastia (or pseudogynaecomastia) is of no use, as an increase in glandular tissue and in fat lead to an identical clinical appearance, even though the relation of fatty and glandular tissue may be different. The male glandular tissue and the surrounding fat of the breast are estrogen-susceptible. Gynaecomastia may occur with an increase of estrogen concentrations at the cellular level, followed by an imbalance of androgen and estrogen action, as is most notable in androgen-receptor defects.

A physiological gynaecomastia is found in the newborn, where it depends on the maternal estrogens; in pubertal boys, where it resolves itself spontaneously; and in aging men. The frequency in the general population is high. Niewöhner and Nuttall (1984) found a gynaecomastia in 65% of men; the percentage was higher in men older than 50 years. In a study with 115 patients of a dermatology department, a gynaecomastia was observed in 32 patients (27.8%) (Seibel et al. 1998).

Another rare cause of gynaecomastia is excessive hyperprolactinemia. It is independent of the cause of hyperprolactinemia, which may be induced by pituitary adenoma or by drugs (Coppola and Cuomo 1998).

Cutaneous Manifestations. Gynaecomastia may be unilateral or bilateral. The term gynaecomastia is used for all types of increased breast volume and increased swelling of the male breast region, irrespective of the consistence and the degree of swelling. There are no generally accepted clinical thresholds to define a swelling as gynaecomastia. Niewöhner et al. (1984) used a horizontal skinfold as a measure, and suggested gynaecomastia if it exceeded 2 cm (Fig. 8.1).

Khan and Blamey (2003) discriminated two forms of gynaecomastia: a lump type and a fatty type. The former is a single, firm, often retro-areolar lump, the latter is a diffused fatty lesion in the whole breast area. The first type is more common in adolescents, the latter in elderly men. The areola may be enlarged and stronger pigmented. Neither the etiology nor the pathological substrate can be suspected from the clinical appearance.

Clinical diagnosis includes medical history. A number of drugs are suspected to cause gynaecomastia. Also, a number of underlying diseases may cause the imbalance of estrogens

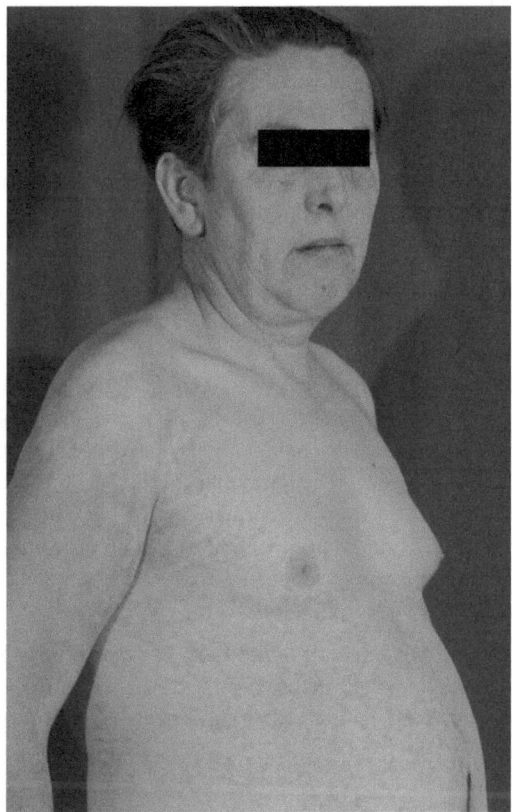

Fig. 8.1 Gynecomastia in a patient with Klinefelter's syndrome

and androgen, and these have to be considered and ruled out by specific diagnostic procedures. The size of the gynaecomastia is confirmed by palpation, measurement of the
diameter of the areola, and a skinfold measurement that includes the swelling.

The size and structure of a breast lump may be described by sonography. The appearance
of a complex cystic mass in the male breast on sonography suggests the possibility of
malignancy, and therefore warrants biopsy (Jun Yang et al. 2002).

Mammography is necessary only in rare cases, when malignancy is not suspected on
clinical grounds (Merkle et al. 1996). Anyhow, the investigation of male breast enlargement
by X-rays appears to be a useful and reliable method.

Fine needle aspirates are suitable to rule out malignancies. In a study, the negative
predictive value and specificity for malignancy was 100%; the positive predictive value
and sensitivity was also 100% (Vetto et al. 1998).

It is important to differentiate benign gynaecomastia from male breast cancer. In general,
the probability that a breast lump in a male breast is a cancer is low. Bilateral breast masses
indicate a low probability of cancer (Volpe et al. 1999). Pain is more common in benign

gynaecomastia, but the lack of symptoms is not helpful in differential diagnosis (Giordano et al. 2002). Gynaecomastia itself is not a risk factor for cancer. Ambrogetti et al. (1996) reported on 748 consecutive male patients, at an average age of 50.5 years, who were referred for breast screening. A malignant lesion was detected in 20 patients (2.67%). Sensitivity for nonmalignancy was high; combined palpation and mammography had 100% sensitivity. The presence of genes that enhance the susceptibility for breast cancer (BRCA-1, BRCA-2, and others) has to be considered (de Jong et al. 2002).

Histopathology. Correct diagnosis is impossible without histological examination of an excided tissue. In the literature, the most frequent differential diagnosis was myofibroblastoma (Magro et al. 2002). Most threatening is the diagnosis of male breast cancer as a cause of breast enlargement.

Williams (1963) described two types of gynaecomastia. Type I, the florid gynaecomastia, is characterized by an increased number of ducts with irregular lumen, in some cases showing pseudolobule formation. The epithelium may have more than three layers, sometimes with small papillae (Fig. 8.2). The ducts may be surrounded by cuffs of connective tissue, which is well demarcated from the normal interlobular connective tissue. Type II, the quiescent gynaecomastia, shows ducts with normal unilayer epithelium, but irregular lumen and slight ectasia. No cuffs of connective tissue are seen. The stroma often shows hyalinization and no fibroblastic proliferation.

Treatment. Pharmacological treatment is of little use. The only drug appearing to be effective is the antiestrogenic compound tamoxifen. It has mostly been used in adolescent gynaecomastia. So far, with respect to possible side effects (liver), the treatment cannot be recommended.

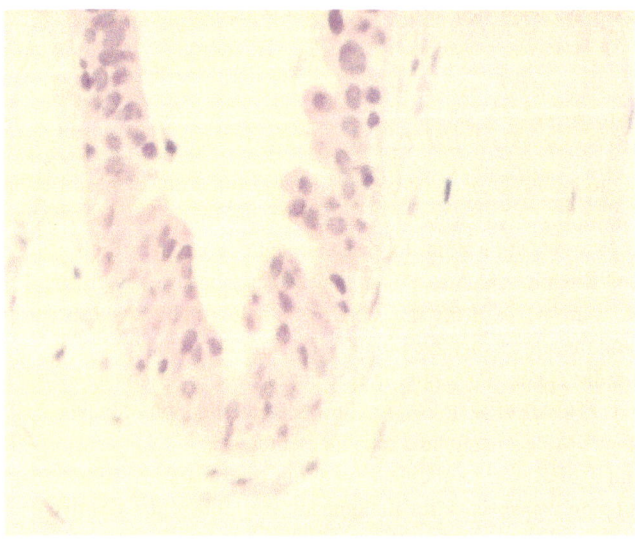

Fig. 8.2 Gynecomastia, histopathology. Normal duct cells in three layers. The duct is surrounded by a cuff of connective tissue

Surgical removal of the enlarged tissue is the treatment of choice. There is a great variety of procedures (Rohrich et al. 2003). Removal through a circumareolar section with purse-string suture is the standard procedure. This creates the best aesthetic results, with few complications or risk of relapse (Persichetti et al. 2001). An alternative surgical procedure in severe gynaecomastia is total mastectomy and free nipple grafting. In recent years, satisfying results were also observed after liposuction.

8.1.2
Skin Diseases of the Male Nipple

Localized Inflammatory Diseases. There are localized infections from nipple piercing, mammillary eczema in allergic contact dermatitis or atopic dermatitis (Fig. 8.3), lymphadenosis benigna cutis, a B-cell lymphoma associated with Borrelia burgdorferi infection, and nevoid hyperkeratosis, which histopathologically resembles the pomade crust observed as a consequence of intense skin care.

Tumors. A number of benign and malignant tumors occur at the nipple. They are listed in Table 8.1.

Malformations. Polythelia is observed in up to 1% of newborns, usually along embryonic milk lines. In most cases, this phenomenon is recognized only during adulthood (Fig. 8.4). A possible association between aberrant mammary tissue and urinary tract malformations is discussed controversially in the literature (Urbani and Betti 1996).

Absence of the nipple occurs in the Finlay-Marjs syndrome (OMIM 181270).

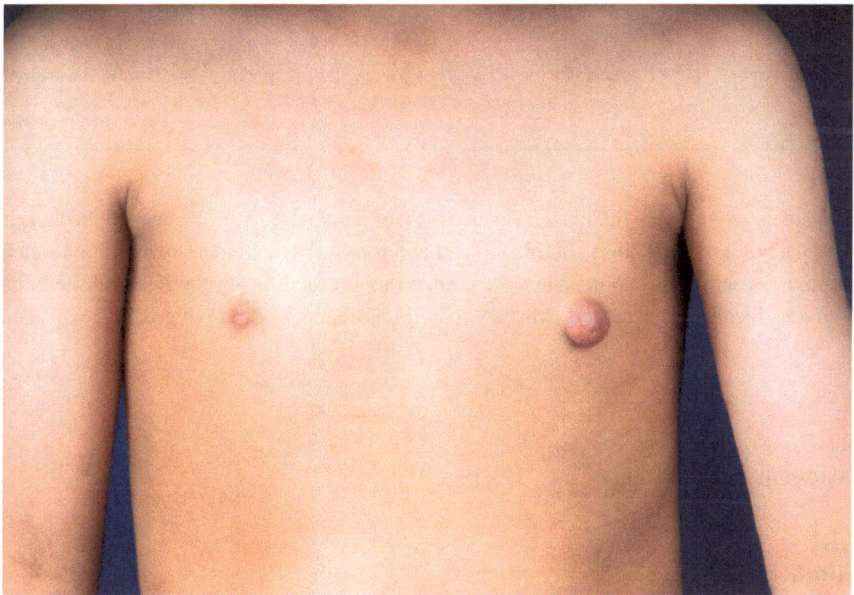

Fig. 8.3 Mamillary eczema in a patient with atopic dermatitis

8

Table 8.1 Tumors of the male nipple

Disease	Clinical appearance	Histopathology	Treatment
Areolar sebaceous hyperplasia (Fig. 8.5)	Whitish or yellowish plaques with papillated surface	Fully differentiated sebaceous glands are observed.	Not known, not necessary
Melanocytic nevi (mole)	Brown, soft papule	Naevus cells (melanocytes)	Excision if desired
Seborrhoic keratosis	Verrucous lesion	Acanthosis, papilloma-tosis, hyperkeratosis	Removal if desired
Skin tags (fibroma pendulans),	Flesh-colored, pedun-culated soft tumor	Folded, acanthotic epidermis, loose connective tissue	Removal if desired
Venous lakes (angioma senile).	Soft, dark-blue papule, easily compressible	Large, jagged vascular space	Removal or coagulation if desired
Leiomyoma	Painless, soft, red papule	Bundles of smooth muscle fibers	Excision if desired
Basal cell carcinoma (BCC)	Asymptomatic, flesh-colored nodule, grows slowly over several months or years	Cell atypia, palisade arrangement of the peripheral cell layer	Excision
Malignant melanoma	Rapidly growing pig-mented tumor, early ulceration	Atypic naevus cells, infiltrating tumor	Excision, assessment of lymph nodes
Paget's disease	Erythematous,	Large, clear cells, immunopositive for ER, CEA, cytokeratin 7. Negative for S-100.	Assessment of underlying breast cancer, stage-dependent treatment
Breast cancer	Swelling of the nipple; carcinoma erysipela-toides	Cell atypia, infiltrating tumor	Excision, assessment of lymph nodes

Surgical Interventions. After bilateral total loss of the nipple due to the treatment of benign and malignant tumors, as well as chronic inflammations or trauma, a reconstruction for aesthetic purposes is useful. It is important to place the new nipple exactly at the physiological site, as has been described by some authors (Murphy et al. 1994; Beer et al. 2001) (Fig. 8.5).

8.2
Estrogens in the Female

8.2.1
Climacteric Skin

Aetiopathogenesis. Estrogens exert direct and indirect effects on the skin. The presence of estrogen receptors α and β was demonstrated in keratinocytes, sebaceous glands,

Fig. 8.4 Supernummerary mamilla (polythelia) localized in the milk line

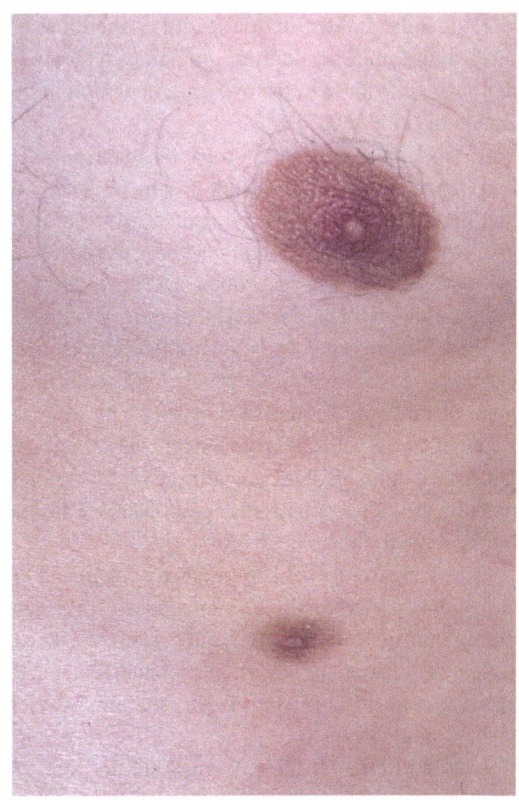

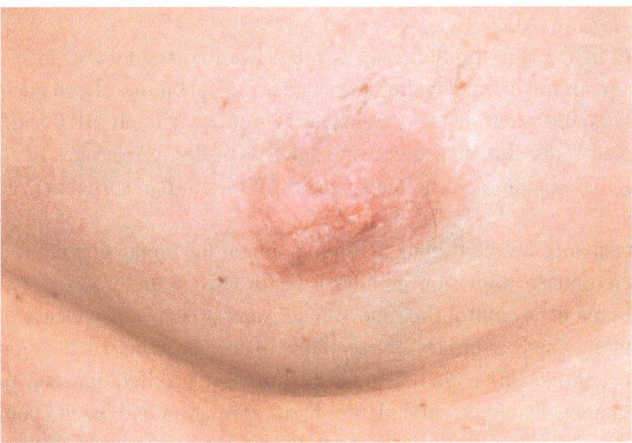

Fig. 8.5 Areolar sebaceous hyperplasia: Whitish and yellowish plaques with papillated surface restricted to the areola

sweat glands, and the dermal papillae, therefore a direct estrogen effect on these structures is possible. In addition, melanocytes express the two estrogen receptors, a fact that may contribute to the hyperpigmentation in hyperestrogenic states (Thornton 2002; Zouboulis et al. 2007).

It was first noticed in 1941 that postmenopausal women had osteoporosis (reduction of bone mass) associated with skin atrophy (reduction of skin thickness). The main constituent that decreases is the collagen content of the skin. An average linear decline of 2.1% of skin collagen and 1.13% skin thickness per postmenopausal year in the initial 15–18 postmenopausal years was described, and the reduction in collagen was closely correlated to years following menopause. The decline in skin collagen content after menopause occurs at a much more rapid rate in the initial postmenopausal years than in the later ones. Skin elasticity also correlates negatively with years since menopause, while hormone replacement therapy (HRT) increases elasticity by 5% over a year (Verdier-Sevrain et al. 2006; Zouboulis et al. 2007). Histological studies and studies using 22.5 MHz ultrasound have indicated a thinning of the epidermis with a loss of rete pegs, i.e. a flattening of the basement membrane with age and after menopause. Estrogen replacement inhibited the thinning (Brincat 2000).

The decrease of both the collagen content and the elasticity contribute to the wrinkles, that appear preferentially on sun-exposed areas. The intensity of the wrinkles depends on various intrinsic factors (heredity, ethnicity, hormonal, and pathological) or extrinsic factors (irradiation, pollution, temperature, and air humidity). Pathohistologically, wrinkles show atrophy of dermal collagen, alterations of elastic fibers, and marked decrease in glycosaminoglycans.

The lipid layer of the epidermis and the skin surface lipids are diminished, resulting in skin dryness. The skin microcirculation is impaired. Blood vessel reactivity in the skin vessels of normal women has been shown to vary over the course of the menstrual cycle. In women on HRT, the nailfold capillary blood flow was shown to increase by 20–30%. However, the autonomic vascular flow (as measured by laser-Doppler flowmetry) in postmenopausal women on long-term HRT was not significantly different when estrogen-treated women were compared to untreated postmenopausal women (Brincat 2000; Raine-Fenning et al. 2003).

The ability of the skin to hold water is related to the stratum corneum lipids, which play a predominant role in maintaining the skin barrier function. A large population-based cohort study demonstrated that postmenopausal women without HRT had significantly higher incidence of dry skin than those using HRT. Transdermal estrogen treatment led to a significant increase in the water-holding capacity of the stratum corneum (Verdier-Sevrain et al. 2006).

Estrogens enhance wound healing by suppression of the production of proinflammatory cytokines, macrophage migration inhibitory factor (MIF), and TNFα by macrophages. Estrogen prevents neutrophil influx into wounds, and prevents the release of neutrophil-derived elastase, which degrades extracellular matrix proteins such as proteoglycans, collagen, and fibronectin. Estradiol induces fibroblast proliferation and production of extracellular matrix, leading to granulation tissue formation and wound contraction. The additional increase in the production of NGF may lead to the enhancement of wound reinnervation and reepithelization (Kanda and Watanabe 2005).

Fig. 8.6 The climacteric skin includes wrinkling, dryness, atrophy, laxity. The changes add to the effects of chronological aging, sunlight exposure, and environmental factors

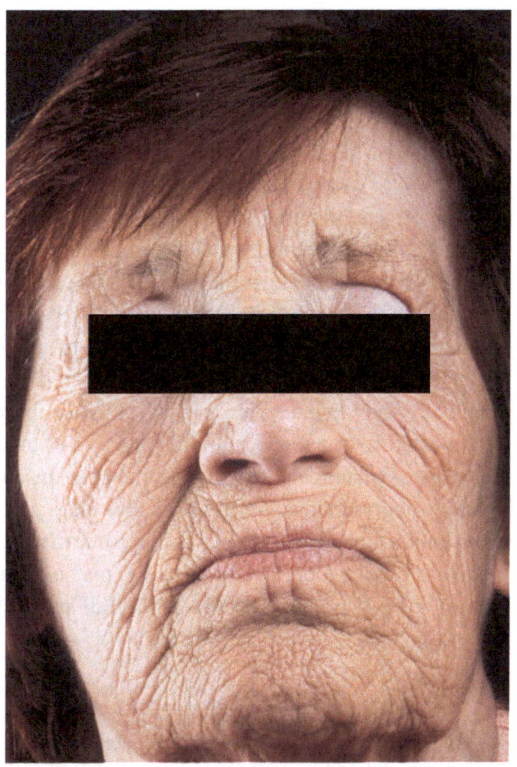

Cutaneous Manifestations. The effects of estrogen deprivation on skin, as present after menopause, include wrinkling (Fig. 8.6), dryness due to changes in the lipid layer of the epidermis and skin surface lipids, atrophy, laxity, poor wound healing, hot flashes, and vulvar atrophy. Estrogen deficiency after menopause leads to changes in the skin biology, in addition to the effects of chronological aging, sunlight exposure, and environmental factors (Hall and Philipps 2005).

Treatment. All the changes appearing in menopause can partly be revised with HRT, but a number of studies also showed that topical administration may exert beneficial effects on the skin or may be even superior to systemic HRT (Oikarinen 2000). The progressive increase in skin extensibility and decrease in elasticity with aging was found to be slowed by the use of HRT. In general, hormone creams have a rich history in cosmetic dermatology. In the 1930s, hormone creams were already the most popular cosmeceutical facial moisturizers in the United States (Draelos 2005). There is currently no other substance available that delivers such documented and reproducible results in women (Brincat et al. 2005), and estradiol is therefore the preferred hormone in studies of "hormonal cosmetics" (Gruber et al. 2002).

In 1997, a large, but uncontrolled, study (Dunn et al. 1997) included 3,875 women aged 40 years and older, who participated in a study on the effect of topical estrogen application on the skin conditions of wrinkling, dryness, and atrophy. The prevalence of all three skin conditions was lower in African American women, compared with white women. Among all women, estrogen use was associated with a statistically significant decrease in the likelihood of senile dry skin (OR 0.76; 95% CI 0.60–0.97) and wrinkling, while it was not associated with skin atrophy.

In addition, several controlled studies have been able to shown that estrogen treatment increases skin collagen or skin thickness (Table 8.2). Studies in nuns helped to differentiate the effects of estrogen deficiency from that of lifetime sun exposure and smoking. After 24 weeks of treatment with estrogen-containing crème, a significant improvement of skin profile and thickness was observed, in comparison to a placebo treatment (Verdier-Sevrain 2007). Another controlled study observed significant reduction of wrinkle depth and increase in skin hydration after estrogen treatment, in comparison to placebo treatment (Sator et al. 2004). In the two studies, no significant side effects were observed. A third controlled study found an increase in epidermal thickness after 6 months.

An increase in the concentration and size of elastic fibers was observed in postmenopausal women applying 2 mg/d of estradiol to the abdomen for 3 weeks. Evaluation of the laxity through noninvasive methods also showed a dependency on estrogen levels. The combination of increased dermal volume (due to more collagen fibers) and increased dermal hydration (due to more hyaluronic acid) may explain the decreased wrinkling apparent in women using estrogens (Draelos 2005; Hall and Philipps 2005).

Table 8.2 Estrogen effects on skin collagen or skin thickness in humans (results from controlled studies) and review of studies evaluating skin collagen content in patients receiving hormone replacement therapy (Hall and Philipps 2005; Verdier-Sevrain et al. 2006)

Study	Type of measurement	Hormones used	Results
Castelo-Branco et al. 1992	Skin biopsy analysis	Conjugated equine estrogens or transdermal 17b-estradiol	Increase in skin collagen of 1.8–5.1% after HRT for 12 months
Callens et al. 1996	Skin thickness measured by ultrasonagraphy	17b-estradiol gel or estradiol patches	Increase in skin thickness of 7–15%
Maheux et al. 1994	Skin thickness measured by ultrasonagraphy	Conjugated estrogen 0.625 mg	Increase in skin thickness by 11.5% after HRT for 12 months
Varila et al. 1995	Skin biopsy analysis	Topical 17b-estradiol	Increase in hydroxyproline by 38% after treatment for 3 months
Sauerbronn et al. 2000	Computerized image analysis of collagen fibers	2 mg estradiol in 21-d cycle, 6 mo	6.5% increase in collagen, medial upper arm
Bolognia et al. 1989	Questionnaire, examination	transdermal 17b-estradiol (50 or 100 µg), 6 mo	no statistical difference in symptoms of dryness, itching, bruising, or thinning of the skin.

Estrogens also have effects on skin pigmentation. An increase of pigmentation is common during pregnancy and during the use of oral contraceptives. There are few reports on the effects of topical estrogen application on pigment changes in photoaged skin. No improvement of dyspigmentation was observed (Verdier-Sevrain et al. 2006).

Even though systemic and topical estrogen application is so effective, adverse effects, not only to the skin but also to other organs, have to be carefully observed. There have been some concerns that estrogens predispose women to malignant melanoma, but the association was not proven. The effects of HRT on the cardiovascular system and the growth of estrogen-dependent tumors should be considered (Draelos 2005).

The legal and medical restrictions on the use of estrogen has led to an interest in phytoestrogens, especially those derived from soy. It has been postulated that isoflavones might confer positive estrogen-like effects with fewer adverse effects. The main groups represent isoflavones and lignans. Estrogenic activity in most phytoestrogens is demonstrated through interaction with the estrogen receptors. Genistein, the most widely studied isoflavone, may have some protective benefit from UV-induced skin damage.

Bayerl and Keil (2002) studied the topical application of phytoestrogens. They found an increase in epidermal and dermal thickness. A controlled, but not comparing, European multicenter study examined the effect of a cosmetic cream preparation in women who were not using HRT, over 12 weeks. Skin dryness and roughness were significantly improved at the treated areas, in comparison with the untreated skin areas. At the end of the treatment period, facial wrinkles were significantly reduced by 22%, and skin looseness was significantly reduced by 24%. Hall and Philipps (2005) studied 202 healthy postmenopausal women aged 60–75 years in a double-blind, randomized, placebo-controlled trial. The women applied soy protein containing 99 mg isoflavones, daily for 12 months, versus placebo. Cognitive function, bone mineral density, and lipid profiles were assessed. After 1 year, there were no differences observed between the active treatment and placebo groups. In another double-blind, placebo-controlled study, the effects of isoflavones on menopausal symptoms, including dry skin, facial hair, libido, and vaginal dryness, were evaluated in 94 postmenopausal women aged 50–75 years. Three months of soy supplements containing phytoestrogens did not provide symptomatic relief, compared with placebo.

8.2.2
Autoimmune Estrogen Dermatitis

The existence of this entity is not generally accepted. The proof that estrogen dermatitis is an autoimmune disease has not yet been met. The hallmark of estrogen dermatitis is the cyclic premenstrual flare. The clinical picture varies. Intradermal tests are necessary to establish the diagnosis. Persistence of a papule for more than 24 h is considered a positive test. Even more convincing is the reactivation of the test site during future premenstrual periods (Shelley et al. 1995). In 1995, more than 30 examples of autoimmune progesterone dermatitis were reported, but only 17 cases of estrogen dermatitis. Each had a positive intradermal skin test to estrone. They showed vesicles on the face with secondary impetiginization. The lesions worsened and new ones appeared premenstrually.

8

In 2003, Yotsumoto et al. reported on 7 patients with estrogen dermatitis, who had red papules, urticaria, as well as acneiform and annular erythema. They had a positive intradermal test with estradiol preparation (10 mg ml^{-1}, diluted 1:100 in saline). It has been shown that estrogen enhanced histamine and serotonin release from human basophils, while they were inhibited by tamoxifen. In addition, eosinophils stimulated by a combination of estrogen and progesterone showed a significant induction of degranulation in nasal mucosa. The histopathology showed nests of mononuclear cells in the epidermis and/or in the hair follicles. Immune histochemical staining showed that most of the mononuclear cells in the nests were CD1a- and CD83-positive Langerhans cells. CD1a- and CD83-positive dendritic cells were distributed in the hair follicles and perifollicular regions, as well as in the epidermis. Lymphocytes were densely gathered in the vicinity of CD1a- and CD83-positive cells, not only in the perifollicular regions, but also in the perivascular regions. Therefore, it seems that a dendritic-cell-mediated allergic mechanism is involved in estrogen dermatitis.

The beneficial effects of tamoxifen were described in the treatment of estrogen dermatitis. Dermatitis induced by both estrogen and progesterone responds to tamoxifen (10 mg per day). Progesterone therapy is also helpful in treating estrogen dermatitis. Oophorectomy is the most radical treatment, but the cure will be permanent (Shelley et al. 1995; Kim et al. 1997)

Recent reports may explain the reason why tamoxifen was effective in patients with estrogen dermatitis. Tamoxifen acts as an immune suppressor by inhibiting the maturation and differentiation of dendritic cells, thus suppressing the antigen-presenting function of Langerhans cells. It is possible that tamoxifen may be useful not only in estrogen dermatitis, but also in cutaneous diseases in which Langerhans cells are activated (Yotsumoto et al. 2003).

8.2.3
Unilateral Nevoid Telangiectasia

Unilateral nevoid teleangiectasia (UNT) was first described by Blaschko in 1899. Since then, about 100 cases have been reported (Hynes and Shenefelt 1997). The feature is associated with hyperestrogenic conditions in females, and with liver cirrhosis in males. The disease in females often occurs along the Blaschko lines; it appears to be caused by somatic mutation inducing localized increase in estrogen susceptibility. Enhanced concentrations of estrogen receptor protein in the cytosol of lesional skin were demonstrated (Uhlin and McCarty 1983). The disease in males may have another pathomechanism.

UNT in women appears frequently in the last trimenon of pregnancy (Greer 1974; Wilkin 1977; Labohm et al. 1985; Uhlin and McCarty 1983). In men, UNT is associated with liver cirrhosis or hepatitis C and B (Jucas et al. 1979; Raff and Bardach 1982; Karakas et al. 2004). In addition, UNT was associated with autoimmune or spinal diseases (Wollina et al. 2001), and was also observed in a healthy adult male (Taskapan et al. 1997). The latter observations, however, are doubtful in the affiliation to the disease.

Clinically, distributed singular teleangiectatic lesions of macular or spider-like appearance are observed. They are restricted to circumscribed areas, predominantly in the upper

Fig. 8.7 Unilateral nevoid
teleangiectasia. Singular teleangiectatic lesions of macular or spider-
like appearance are restricted to
circumscribed areas, predominantly
in the upper trunk and arms of only
one side of the body

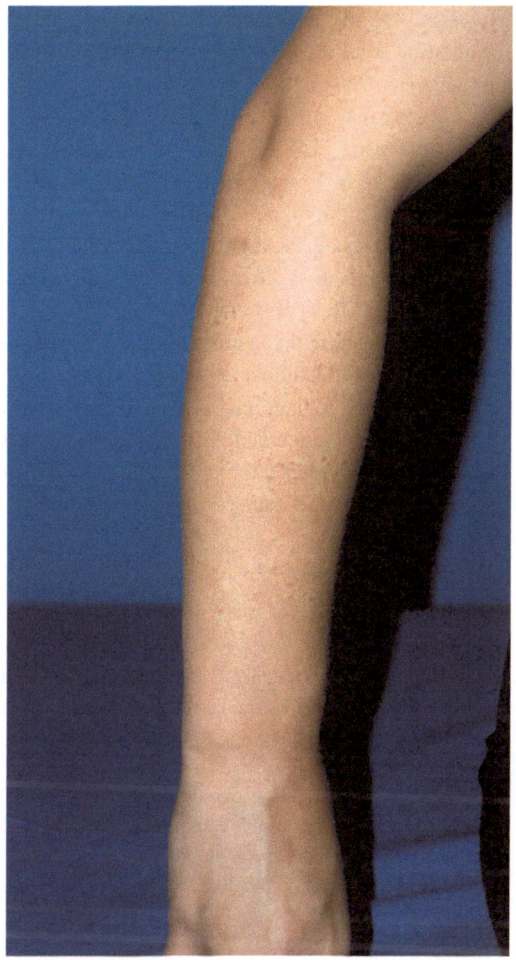

trunk and arms of only one side of the body (Fig. 8.7). There are no subjective symptoms.
Histopathologic examination shows only dilated vascular structures, without inflammatory
infiltration.

Treatment of UNT is possible with laser light (Henry et al. 2006).

8.2.4
Melanoma and Estrogens

Estrogen receptors are present in some skin tumors, as demonstrated by both histochemical
and biochemical assays. Cutaneous melanoma cytosol contains a high-affinity low-capacity
receptor for estrogen. The application of estradiol, progesterone, and dihydrotestosterone
to melanoma cells in vitro induced an inhibition of 3H-thymidine uptake in those cells

expressing the respective hormone receptor. The growth inhibition was counteracted by the addition of interleukin-8, but only in those expressing the respective receptor (Kanda and Watanabe 2001).

Estrogens play a role in melanocyte metabolism, but melanoma is not an estrogen-dependent tumor. The determination of estrogen receptor status is not useful in the management of malignant melanomas. As melanoma has a significantly better prognosis in women than in men, an influence of steroid hormones is likely. Hormone receptors for estrogens, progestogens, androgens, and glucocorticoids were demonstrated in more than half of the melanomas investigated, but only a small percentage responded to hormonal manipulation, such as the treatment with the estrogen antagonist tamoxifen (Neifeld 1996). It is thus unclear whether estrogens or androgens are responsible for the differences in the clinical cause of melanoma (Rampen 1984).

It appears that melanoma cannot be regarded as a contraindication for HRT. Although some authors advise avoidance of HRT in the first 2 years after the diagnosis of melanoma, there is no clear evidence for an influence of HRT on the course of the disease (Durvasula et al. 2002; Leslie and Espey 2005).

References

Ambrogetti D, Ciatto S, Catarzi S, Muraca MG. The combined diagnosis of male breast lesions: a review of a series of 748 consecutive cases. Radiol Med (Torino). 1996;91(4):356–9.

Bayerl C, Keil D. Isoflavonoide in der Behandlung der Hautalterung postmenopausaler Frauen. Akt Dermatol. 2002;28:14–18.

Beer GM, Budi S, Seifert B, Morgenthaler W, Infanger M, Meyer VE. Configuration and localization of the nipple-areola complex in men. Plast Reconstr Surg. 2001;108(7):1947–52

Brincat MP. Hormone replacement therapy and the skin. Maturitas. 2000;35(2):107–17.

Brincat MP, Baron YM, Galea R. Estrogens and the skin. Climacteric. 2005;8(2):110–23.

Callens A, Valliant L, Lecomte P, et al. Does hormonal skin aging exist? A study of the influence of different hormone therapy regimens on the skin of postmenopausal women using non-invasive measurement techniques. Dermatology 1996;193:289–94.

Castelo-Branco C, Duran M, Gonzales-Merlo J. Skin collagen and bone changes related to age and hormone replacement therapy. Maturitas 1992;14:113–9.

Coppola A, Cuomo MA. Prolactinoma in the male. Physiopathological, clinical, and therapeutic features. Minerva Endocrinol. 1998;23(1):7–16.

de Jong MM, Nolte IM, te Meerman GJ, van der Graaf WT, Oosterwijk JC, Kleibeuker JH, Schaapveld M, de Vries EG. Genes other than BRCA1 and BRCA2 involved in breast cancer susceptibility. J Med Genet. 2002;39(4):225–42.

Draelos ZD. Topical and oral estrogens revisited for antiaging purposes. Fertil Steril. 2005;84(2):291–2

Dunn LB, Damesyn M, Moore AA, Reuben DB, Greendale GA. Does estrogen prevent skin aging? Results from the First National Health and Nutrition Examination Survey (NHANES I). Arch Dermatol. 1997;133(3):339–42.

Durvasula R, Ahmed SM, Vashisht A, Studd JW. Hormone replacement therapy and malignant melanoma: to prescribe or not to prescribe? Climacteric. 2002;5(2):197–200.

Giordano SH, Buzdar AU, Hortobagyi GN. Breast cancer in men. Ann Intern Med. 2002;137(8):678–87.

Greer KE. Letter: unilateral nevoid telangiectasia. Arch Dermatol. 1974;109(1):100–1.

Gruber CJ, Wieser F, Gruber IM, Ferlitsch K, Gruber DM, Huber JC. Current concepts in aesthetic endocrinology. Gynecol Endocrinol. 2002;16(6):431–41.

Hall G, Phillips TJ. Estrogen and skin: the effects of estrogen, menopause, and hormone replacement therapy on the skin. J Am Acad Dermatol. 2005;53(4):555–68; quiz 569–72.

Henry F, Quatresooz P, Valverde-Lopez JC, Piérard GE. Blood vessel changes during pregnancy: a review. Am J Clin Dermatol. 2006;7(1):65–9.

Hynes LR, Shenefelt PD. Unilateral nevoid telangiectasia: occurrence in two patients with hepatitis C. J Am Acad Dermatol. 1997;36(5 Pt 2):819–22.

Jucas JJ, Rietschel RL, Lewis CW. Unilateral nevoid telangiectasia. Arch Dermatol. 1979; 115(3):359–60.

Jun Yang Y. Gynecomastia with marked cellular atypia associated with chemotherapy. Arch Pathol Lab Med. 2002;126(5):613–4.

Kanda N, Watanabe S. 17beta-estradiol, progesterone, and dihydrotestosterone suppress the growth of human melanoma by inhibiting interleukin-8 production. J Invest Dermatol. 2001;117(2):274–83.

Kanda N, Watanabe S. Regulatory roles of sex hormones in cutaneous biology and immunology. J Dermatol Sci. 2005;38(1):1–7.

Karakaş M, Durdu M, Sönmezo lu S, Akman A, Gümürdülü D. Unilateral nevoid telangiectasia. J Dermatol. 2004;31(2):109–12.

Khan HN, Blamey KW. Edocrine treatment of physiological gynaecomastia. Tamoxifen seems to be effective. BMJ 2003;327:301–302

Kim KH, Yoon TJ, Oh CW, Kim TH. A case of estrogen dermatitis. J Dermatol. 1997;24(5):332–6.

Labohm EB, Miseré JF, Veen C. Unilaterales nävoides Telangiektasie-Syndrom. Hautarzt. 1985;36(2):107–8.

Leslie KK, Espey E. Oral contraceptives and skin cancer: is there a link? Am J Clin Dermatol. 2005;6(6):349–55.

Magro G, Gurrera A, Scavo N, Lanzafame S, Bisceglia M. Fibromatosis of the breast: a clinical, radiological and pathological study of 6 cases. Pathologica. 2002 Oct;94(5):238–46.

Maheux R, Naud F, Rioux M, et al. A randomized, double-blind, placebo-controlled study on the effect of conjugated estrogens on skin thickness. Am J Obstet Gynecol 1994;170:642–9.

Merkle E, Muller M, Vogel J, Klatt S, Gorich J, Beger HG, Brambs HJ. Clinical relevance of mammography in men. Rofo Fortschr Geb Rontgenstr Neuen Bildgeb Verfahr. 1996;164(1):7–12.

Murphy TP, Ehrlichman RJ, Seckel BR. Nipple placement in simple mastectomy with free nipple grafting for severe gynecomastia. Plast Reconstr Surg. 1994;94(6):818–23.

Neifeld JP. Endocrinology of melanoma. Semin Surg Oncol. 1996;12(6):402–6.

Niewöhner CB, Nuttall RQ:Gynecomastia in a hospitalized male population. Am J Med (1984);77:633–8.

Oikarinen A. Systemic estrogens have no conclusive beneficial effect on human skin connective tissue. Acta Obstet Gynecol Scand. 2000;79(4):250–4.

Persichetti P, Berloco M, Casadei RM, Marangi GF, Di Lella F, Nobili AM. Gynecomastia and the complete circumareolar approach in the surgical management of skin redundancy. Plast Reconstr Surg. 2001;107(4):948–54.

Raff M, Bardach HG. Unilaterales nävoides Telangiektasiesyndrom. Hautarzt. 1982;33(3): 148–51.

Raine-Fenning NJ, Brincat MP, Muscat-Baron Y. Skin aging and menopause: implications for treatment. Am J Clin Dermatol. 2003;4(6):371–8.

Rampen FH. Sex differences in survival from cutaneous melanoma. Int J Dermatol. 1984;23(7): 444–52.

Rohrich RJ, Ha RY, Kenkel JM, Adams WP Jr. Classification and management of gynecomastia: defining the role of ultrasound-assisted liposuction. Plast Reconstr Surg. 2003;111(2):909–23.

Sator PG, Schmidt JB, Rabe T, Zouboulis CC. Skin aging and sex hormones in women – clinical perspectives for intervention by hormone replacement therapy. Exp Dermatol. 2004;13(Suppl 4):36–40.

Sauerbronn AVD, Fonseca AM, Bagnoli VR, et al. The effects of systemic hormone replacement therapy on the skin of the postmenopausal women. Int J Gynecol Obstet 2000;68:35–41.

Seibel V, Müller HH, Krause W. Die Inzidenz der Gynäkomastie bei dermatologischen Patienten. Hautarzt 1998;49:382–7.

Shelley WB, Shelley ED, Talanin NY, Santoso-Pham J. Estrogen dermatitis. J Am Acad Dermatol. 1995;32(1):25–31.

Taşkapan O, Harmanyeri Y, Sener O, Aksu A. Acquired unilateral nevoid telangiectasia syndrome. Acta Derm Venereol. 1997;77(1):62–3.

Thornton MJ. The biological actions of estrogens on skin. Exp Dermatol. 2002;11(6):487–502.

Uhlin SR, McCarty KS Jr. Unilateral nevoid telangiectatic syndrome. The role of estrogen and progesterone receptors. Arch Dermatol. 1983;119(3):226–8.

Urbani CE, Betti R. Accessory mammary tissue associated with congenital and hereditary neph-rourinary malformations. Int J Dermatol. 1996;35(5):349–52.

Varila E, Rantala I, Oikarinen A, et al. The effect of topical oestradiol on skin collagen of postmenopausal women. Br J Obstet Gynaecol 1995;120(12):985–9.

Verdier-Sevrain S. Effect of estrogens on skin aging and the potential role of selective estrogen receptor modulators. Climacteric. 2007;10(4):289–97.

Verdier-Sevrain S, Bonte F, Gilchrest B. Biology of estrogens in skin: implications for skin aging. Exp Dermatol. 2006;15(2):83–94.

Vetto J, Schmidt W, Pommier R, DiTomasso J, Eppich H, Wood W, Moseson D. Accurate and cost-effective evaluation of breast masses in males. Am J Surg. 1998;175(5):383–7.

Volpe CM, Raffetto JD, Collure DW, Hoover EL, Doerr RJ. Unilateral male breast masses: cancer risk and their evaluation and management. Am Surg. 1999;65(3):250–3.

Wilkin JK. Unilateral nevoid telangiectasia: three new cases and the role of estrogen. Arch Dermatol. 1977;113(4):486–8.

Williams MJ. Gynecomastia. Its incidenc, recognition and host characteization in 447 autopsy cases. Am J Med. 1963;34:103–12.

Wollina U, Barta U, Uhlemann C, Oelzner P. Acquired nevoid telangiectasia. Dermatology. 2001;203(1):24–6.

Yotsumoto S, Shimomai K, Hashiguchi T, Uchimiya H, Usuki K, Nishi M, Kanekura T, Kanzaki T. Estrogen dermatitis: a dendritic-cell-mediated allergic condition. Dermatology. 2003;207:265–8

Zouboulis CC, Chen WC, Thornton MJ, Qin K, Rosenfield R. Sexual hormones in human skin. Horm Metab Res. 2007;39(2):85–95.

Gestagens

Synopsis

Pregnancy Dermatoses

> Specific dermatoses of pregnancy are of unknown aetiology. The most frequent dermatosis of pregnancy are pruritic urticarial papules and plaques of pregnancy (PUPPP). They occur predominantly in the third trimenon. In rare cases, they have also been observed outside pregnancy. For treatment, external or even systemic glucocorticoids are recommended and the prognosis is good.

> Atopic eczema in pregnancy (AEP) is the most common pruritic condition in pregnancy, seen in almost 50% of patients. Skin lesions start commonly during early pregnancy. Lesio.ns comprise features and distribution of chronic eczema with lichenfication, vesiculous and pruriginous papules together with intense pruritus. For treatment, external glucocorticoids are used.

> Pemphigoid gestationis (PG) is rare. Epidermal basement membrane zone antibodies are present in serum, binding to the 180-kD antigen of bullous pemphigoid. Patients experience abrupt onset of an intensely pruritic urticarial lesion in the second or third trimester. The antibodies may be transferred to the foetus, so that the newborn suffers from similar cutaneous lesions. For treatment, systemic glucocorticoids are used.

> Pigmentation disorders are common in pregnancy affecting up to 50–70% of women. Higher incidence of chloasma gravidarum or melasma occurs in women with skin type III or higher. Genetic and environmental factors, in particular UV exposure, contribute to intensity of chloasma.

> General skin diseases may occur incidentally in pregnancy. It remains to be clarified whether the incidence is higher than in a comparable time period of women of similar age; satisfying statistical comparisons are not available in literature. 60–88% of women develop striae during pregnancy. Risk factors are: family history of striae in the mother, baseline and delivery body mass index, and striae reported outside the pregnancy.

Continued

Walter K. H. Krause, *Cutaneous Manifestations of Endocrine Diseases*,
DOI: 10.1007/978-3-540-88367-8, © Springer-Verlag Berlin Heidelberg 2009

9

Synopsis *Continued*

> Pregnancy and skin tumours: Lack of immune rejection of the embryo and foetus is based on site-specific immunosuppression at the foetal–maternal interface, but the peripheral immune response of the mother is uninhibited. Earlier, it was a doctrine that a woman who had melanoma should not become pregnant. In some series, women who were pregnant at the time of diagnosis exhibited unfavourable survival prospects. More recent studies, have however refuted this suggestion. The monitoring of nevi in pregnancy has also failed to reveal any reliable changes.

Autoimmune Progesterone Dermatitis

Autoimmune progesterone dermatitis is a rare disease. The aetiopathogenesis remains unclear; the autoimmune origin is not sufficiently proven. The features of autoimmune progesterone dermatitis include eczema, purpura, erythema multiforme, and urticaria. Histopathologically, the skin lesions are usually described as an eosinophilic non-specific vasculitis. For diagnosis, eruptions 7 days before menses and resolving after 1–3 days thereafter as well as positive skin test to progesterone are essential. Treatment of current troubles requires antihistamines and/or glucocorticoids, but the inhibition of endogenous progesterone secretion is essential.

9.1
Pregnancy Dermatoses

9.1.1
Specific Dermatoses of Pregnancy

Aetiopathogenesis. According to Holmes and Black (1983), pemphigus gestationis (PG) (syn. herpes gestationis), pruritic urticarial papules and plaques of pregnancy (PUPPP) (syn. polymorphic eruption of pregnancy [PEP]), and pruritic folliculitis of pregnancy (PF) are acknowledged as specific dermatoses of pregnancy. Their aetiology is still unknown (Nilles et al. 1989; Elling et al. 2000; Matz et al. 2006). Placental products, hormonal alterations, damage to connective tissue with subsequent conversion of non-antigenic structures to antigens are considered to be pathogenic factors (Vaughan Jones et al. 1999; Sherard and Atkinson 2001). Presence of male DNA in the skin lesion has also been reported. No known major autoimmune background played a part in the pathogenesis of the disease (Alcalay et al. 1988). Sex hormone levels in serum in patients with PUPPP showed no significant differences from unaffected pregnant controls.

Cutaneous Manifestations. Lesions of pregnancy dermatoses are characteristic, but not specific in a narrower sense. Table 9.1 summarizes clinical symptoms and diagnostic criteria.

Based on the observations in 401 pregnant patients, Ambros-Rudolph et al. (2006) proposed a slightly divergent classification of the specific dermatoses of pregnancy as given in

Table 9.1 Diagnostic criteria for pregnancy dermatoses (Vaughan Jones et al. 1999)

Pregnancy dermatosis	Diagnostic criteria
Polymorphic eruption of pregnancy	Papulovesicular or urticarial eruption on trunk and limbs with negative immunofluorescence
Pruritic folliculitis of pregnancy	Follicular or pustular (acneiform) eruption with negative immunofluorescence
Prurigo of pregnancy (of Besnier)	Excoriated nodules on trunk/limbs
Pemphigoid gestationis	Bullous eruption: linear deposition of C3 at the basement membrane zone-IgG on immunofluorescence

Table 9.2 Specific dermatoses of pregnancy ($n = 401$). Data gives absolute numbers and percentages (in paranthesis). (From Ambros-Rudolph et al. 2006)

Group	PG ($n = 21$)	PUPPP ($n = 109$)	AEP ($n = 256$)	ICP ($n = 15$)
Primigravidae	10 (48)	79 (73)	113 (44)	7 (47)
Multiple gestation pregnancy	0	17 (16)	2 (1)	0
Previously affected pregnancies	1/11 (9)	2/30 (7)	48/140 (34)	7/8 (88)
Onset before third trimester	6 (29)	3 (3)	191 (75)	3 (20)
Mean onset (range), weeks of gestation	14–38	17–41	2–39	24–36
Localization: abdominal involvement	20 (95)	107 (98)	173 (68)	5 (36)

AEP, Atopic eruption of pregnancy; ICP, intrahepatic cholestasis of pregnancy; PUPPP, pruritic and urticarial papules and plaques of pregnancy; PG, pemphigoid gestationi

Table 9.2. The term atopic eruption of pregnancy (AEP) covered all patients formerly diagnosed with eczema and pruritic folliculitis in pregnancy and prurigo of pregnancy. They also concluded that another disease, intrahepatic cholestasis of pregnancy (ICP) may have to be omitted from the list of pregnancy dermatoses, as it is not a primary dermatosis but associated with only secondary skin lesions caused by scratching when there is a disturbance of liver function and increase of serum bile acids. All authors agree that PG, PEP, and AEP are distinct entities with stereotypic immune pathologic, clinical, or laboratory findings (Ambros-Rudolph et al. 2006).

The course of the pregnancy and the prognosis for the newborn remains usually unaffected by pregnancy dermatoses. The relation of observed and expected birth weight in these cases was not significantly different from that in pregnancies without dermatoses;[i] the proportion of male infants was higher, but the value did not reach statistical significance (Table 9.3; Vaughan Jones et al. 1999).

PUPPP. The most frequent dermatosis of pregnancy is known as pruritic urticarial papules and plaques of pregnancy (PUPPP) in American literature and as polymorphic

Table 9.3 Outcome of pregnancy after dermatoses of pregnancy (Vaughan Jones et al. 1999)

Diagnosis	No. of cases	Multiple pregnancies	IBR mean (95%-con-fidence interval)	Significance level p of difference to normal	Male infants
Eczema (=AEP)	72	0	0.960 (0.92–1.00)	0.55	54% (of 37)
Pruritic follicu-litis (=AEP)	14	0	0.921 (0.86–0.98)	0.02	70% (of 10)
Prurigo	12	0	0.994 (0.91–1.08)	0.87	63% (of 8)
Polymorphic eruption of pregnancy (=PUPPP)	44	7	1.10 (0.92–1.11)	0.81	67% (of 43)
Pemphigoid gestationis (PG)	15	0	0.819 (0.64–1.00)	0.04	42% (of 12)
Intrahepatic cholestasis (ICP)	4	0	0.872 (0.82–0.94)	0.58	0
Miscellaneous dermatoses	39	0	1.017 (0.93–1.10)	0.67	68% (of 22)

IBR. observed/expected birthweight

eruption of pregnancy (PEP) in British literature. It was first described by Lawley et al. in 1979, who also introduced the term PUPPP.

PUPPP has an incidence of 1 in 160 to 1 in 200 pregnancies. Relapses during subsequent pregnancies are usual. In 159,197 deliveries, PUPPP complicated 42 (0.03%) pregnancies (Ohel et al. 2006; Sheiner et al. 2006). Using a multivariate analysis, the following conditions were found to be significantly associated with PUPPP: multiple pregnancies (OR = 4.9, 95% CI 1.7–14.1), hypertensive disorders (OR = 2.2, 95% CI 1.1–4.7), and induction of labor (OR = 7.6, 95% CI 4.0–14.5). Higher rates of 5-min Apgar scores lower than 7 (OR = 8.0, 95% CI 4.4–14.9) and caesarean deliveries (OR = 2.9, 95% CI 1.5–5.6) were found in the PUPPP as compared to the comparison group. Other perinatal outcome parameters such as oligohydramnion, intrauterine growth restriction, meconium-stained amniotic fluid and perinatal mortality were not associated with occurrence of PUPPP. No significant differences were noted between the groups regarding perinatal outcomes. In a study published by Elling et al. (2000), the rate of PUPPP in single pregnancies was 1 in 200 (0.5%). Multiple pregnancies were at a higher risk of developing PUPPP with 2.9% of twin and 14% of triplet pregnancies affected. Among the 30 PUPPP cases studied by Cohen et al. (1989) three were twin pregnancies (10%), while twin gestation rate at the institution was 1.6%.

PUPPP occurs most commonly in the third trimester. Typically, eruptions begin on the abdomen, often within pre-existing striae, and spread to the thighs and extremities (Fig. 9.1). Involvement of face, palms and soles is unusual (High et al. 2005). Patients experience intensely pruritic urticarial and papular lesions. 75–85% of patients with PUPPP are primigravidas. There are no typical laboratory findings.

Fig. 9.1 PUPPP: Eruptions begin on the abdomen, often within preexisting striae, and spread to the thighs and extremities. Patients experience intensely pruritic urticarial and papular lesions

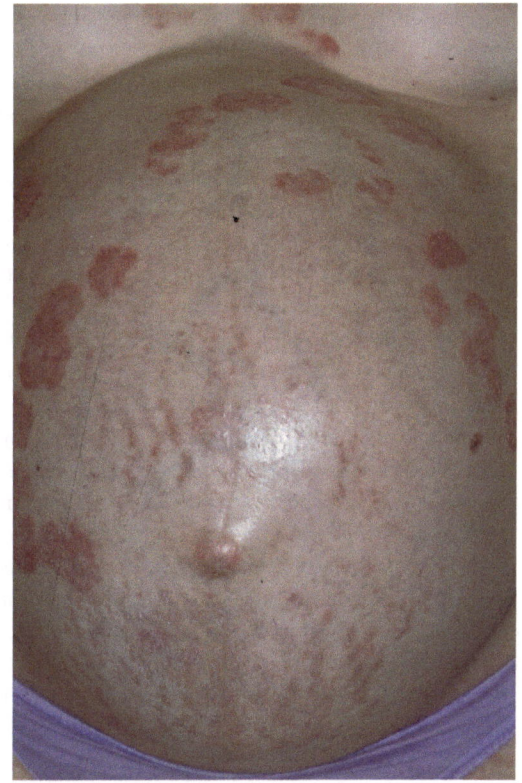

Multiple case reports on unusual cases are found in subject literature. Uhlin (1981) reported on the occurrence of PUPPP in mother and infant. Weiss and Hull (1992) observed two sisters, who were pregnant at the same time, and suffered from PUPPP. They were married to brothers. Two other sisters with PUPPP, pregnant at the same time, were also married to brothers, who were identical twins. The authors were of the view that the mothers shared a genetic susceptibility to develop PUPPP. In addition, a paternal antigen present in the foetal component of the placenta could be released in late pregnancy. A case report of PUPPP beginning 10 days postpartum was published by Buccolo and Viera (2005). MEDLINE searches of literature from 1966 to 2003 made by these authors using the keywords pruritic urticarial papules and plaques of pregnancy or polymorphic eruption of pregnancy and postpartum revealed only two other cases developing in the postpartum period.

Histopathologically, early lesions are accompanied by oedema of the epidermis and papillary dermis, and perivascular lymphocytic infiltrates with variable eosinophils. The density of the infiltrate varies from mild to dense and occasionally extends to deeper levels in the mid-dermis. Advanced lesions may show epidermal changes including focal spongiosis with vesiculation and parakeratosis (Sherard and Atkinson 2001).

The most relevant differential diagnoses are urticaria, hypersensitivity reactions and pemphigoid gestationis. For urticaria, presence of neutrophils can be a diagnostic clue. Hypersensitivity reactions can only be distinguished by the patient's history and clinical presentation. For discrimination of pemphigoid gestationis, immune fluorescence studies are useful and usually reveal negative results in PUPPP (see below). Linear or granular basement membrane staining has been reported in PUPPP, but the intensity is lesser than that found in pemphigoid gestationis (Aronson et al. 1998). Also circulating antibodies against IgM are absent (Zurn et al. 1992). Further, lesions similar to arthropod bites with interstitial eosinophils have been described, but they can be discriminated by the absence of a wedge shaped, deep extending infiltrate, typicalfor arthropod bites.

For the treatment of this disease, external or even systemic glucocorticoids are recommended (Nilles et al. 1989; Sherard and Atkinson 2001). The prognosis is good, since most of the lesions spontaneously resolve within a few days after parturition.

AEP: Ambros-Rudolph et al. (2006) recommended the use of this term, as they found no clear separation between features of eczema in pregnancy, pruritic folliculitis in pregnancy and prurigo of pregnancy. In their study, AEP was the most common pruritic condition in pregnancy, seen in almost 50% of patients. Only 20% of patients with AEP suffered from exacerbation of a pre-existing atopic dermatitis. Skin lesions started commonly during early pregnancy, 36% occurring in the first trimester and onset in 40% of patients in the second trimester. An atopic disposition was demonstrable in about 20% of patients. Lesions comprised features and distribution of chronic eczema with lichenfication, vesiculous and pruriginous papules together with intense pruritus (Fig. 9.2).

The treatment was similar to that used in PUPPP.

Pemphigoid gestationis, originally designated as 'herpes gestationis', is associated with pregnancies, but can also be found in patients with trophoblastic diseases. The incidence is estimated as 1 in 1,700 pregnancies (Roger et al. 1994). It recurs in up to 95% of subsequent pregnancies. Epidermal basement membrane zone antibodies are present in serum, binding to the 180-kD antigen of bullous pemphigoid, a trans-membrane protein within the hemidesmosome. Clinically, patients experience an abrupt onset of an intensely pruritic urticarial lesion in the second or third trimester. Initially, the cutaneous findings are

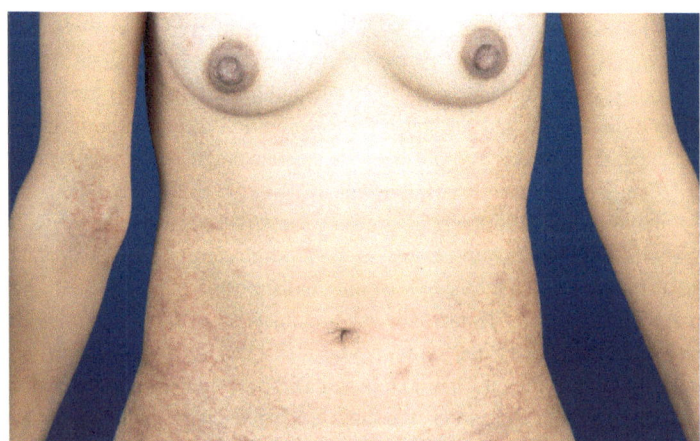

Fig. 9.2 Atopic eczema in pregnancy. Lesions comprise features and distribution of chronic eczema with lichenfication, vesiculous and pruriginous papules together with intense pruritus

limited to the trunk, but later it spreads and spares only the face, palms, soles, and mucous membranes. Up to 25% of the reported cases have been in the immediate postpartum period. The course of the disease in up to 75% of patients is characterized by a spontaneous resolution,late in gestation.In majority of the cases, the disease regresses spontaneously with delivery, although exacerbation might be delayed until 24–48 h after delivery. The antibodies may be transferred to the foetus, in which case the newborn suffers from similar cutaneous lesions (Fig. 9.3). Postpartum flares can be severe and last from weeks to months (Sherard and Atkinson 2001).

Histopathologically. a focal (eosinophilic) spongiosis in the epidermis,and in more developed lesions, necrotic keratinocytes with vacuolar degeneration of the basal layer might occur. In vesiculo-bullous lesions,subepidermal blisters with large numbers of eosinophils and some neutrophils are visible. Early lesions exhibit marked oedema of the papillary dermis and predominant perivascular infiltrate of lymphocytes, histiocytes and numerous eosinophils in the mid-dermis. The infiltrate often lines up along the epidermo-dermal junction (Jolliffe and Sim-Davis 1977). Leukocytoclastic vasculitis and eosinophil dermal papillary micro-abscesses are a rare feature (Daniels and Quadra-White 1981; Laskaris and Angelopoulos 1981). Through immune fluorescence, C3 and sometimes IgG have been demonstrated in a linear arrangement along the basement membrane in lesional and perilesional skin. Using salt split skin,the immune reactants have been localized in the epidermal part within the lamina lucida.

The differentiation of other bullous dermatoses such as epidermolysis bullosa aquisita, dermatitis herpetiformis, linear IgA dermatosis and bullous systemic lupus

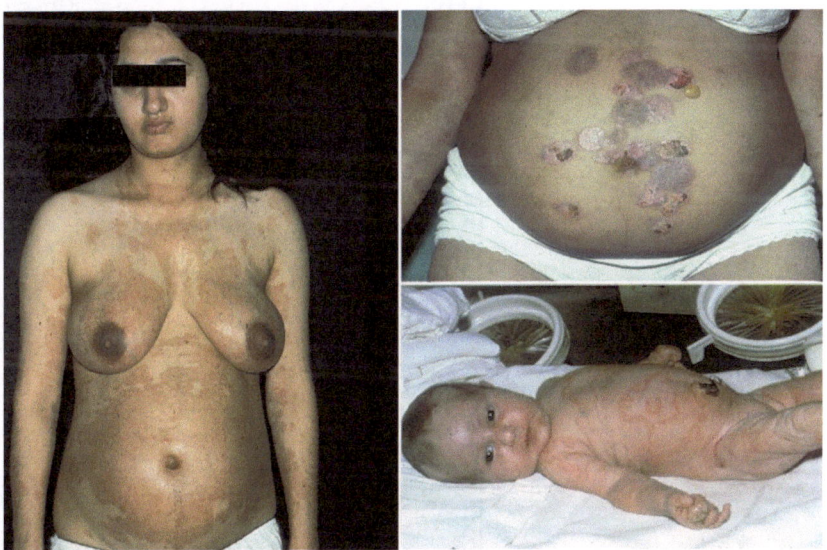

Fig. 9.3 Pemphigoid gestationis. Initially, the bullous lesions are limited to the trunk, but then spreads sparing only the face, palms, soles, and mucous membranes. The bullae pass into erosions, which heal without scarring. The auto-antibodies responsible may be transferred to the foetus, so that the newborn may suffer from similar cutaneous lesions (Courtesy of Prof. M. Hertl, Marburg)

erythematosus is possible only in combination with clinical information and immune fluorescence studies.

For treatment, the regimen published for autoimmune bullous dermatoses including systemic glucocorticoids and immunapheresis have to be considered (Hertl 2005).

9.1.2
Pigmentation Disorders

Cutaneous Manifestations. During pregnancy, significant modifications of pigmentation occur. The most common disorder is chloasma gravidarum, or melasma where the incidence is higher in women with skin type III or higher. It can affect up to 50–70% of pregnant women – Muzaffar et al. (1998) observed increased pigmentation in 90.7% of 140 cases and chloasma in 46.4%. Chloasma also occurs spontaneously during administration of oral contraceptives. Genetic and environmental factors, in particular UV exposure, contribute to the intensity of chloasma.

The pigmentation – diffuse brown hyperpigmentation- is localized on the forehead, cheeks and chin (Fig. 9.4). Increase of pigmentation also concerns nevi and other pigmented lesions. Petraglia et al. (2007) studied the pigment nevi on 35 healthy pregnant women and 35 age-matched female controls. The total number of nevi included was 204. Variables were

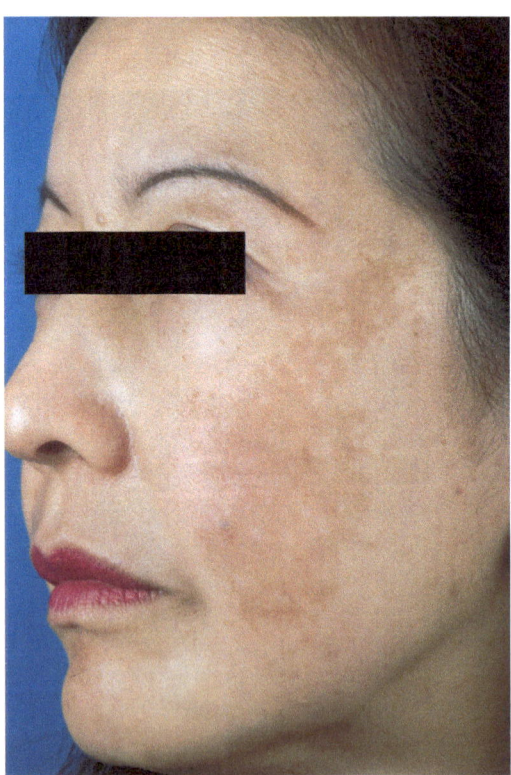

Fig. 9.4 Chloasma. Patchy pigmentation on the forehead is only weak due to the underlying skin type II

measured initially at a particular time (TIME 0) and 12 months after delivery (TIME 2) and in controls, 21 months later, resp. In comparison to the controls, significant modifications in pigmented lesions, especially with regard to pigment network, globules and architectural order–disorder were observed after pregnancy in healthy pregnant women. Obviously, these changes are of little value for the description of melanoma risk in relation to pregnancy.

Zampino et al. (2006) evaluated dermoscopic parameters and total dermoscopic score according to the ABCD rule, and sizes of the nevi in pregnant women. Progressive lightening of the nevi resulted at the end of pregnancy and after delivery occurred. The pigment network showed progressive reduction in prominence and thickness, with increased vessels. At the end of pregnancy a higher total dermoscopic score was observed, with significant reduction in both after delivery. The area did not change significantly. It should be underlined that the changes concern only pigmentation of nevi, but pregnancy is not associated with any significant change in the size of melanocytic nevi (Zampetti et al. 2006).

Treatment. Treatment is summarized in Table 2.5. The use of sunscreens effectively prevents development of chloasma and other pigmentations in pregnant women (Lakhdar et al. 2007).

9.1.3
General Skin Diseases and Striae Gravidarum

General skin diseases may occur incidentally in pregnancy. It remains to be clarified whether the incidence is higher than in a comparable time period of women of similar age; satisfactory statistical comparisons are not available in literature. Vaughan Jones et al. (1999) described the following skin diseases during pregnancy among 200 women: urticaria (7 patients), pityriasis rosea (4 patients), cutaneous lupus erythematosus (3 patients), psoriasis (3 patients), acne vulgaris (3 patients) and lichen planus (2 patients). The incidence appears to be higher than in a comparable population of non-pregnant women, but a reliable comparison has not been identified.

Kumari et al. (2007) studied skin changes in 607 pregnant women. 303 of them were primigravida and 304 were multigravida. The skin diseases observed and the influence of pregnancy are listed in Table 9.4. Physiological changes in pregnancy were observed in 92% as hyperpigmentation and in 80% as striae gravidarum.

Seeger et al. (2007) used data from approximately 2.4 million women aged 10 through 49 years as obtained from health insurance claims to identify whether psoriasis, atopic dermatitis, other inflammatory skin disorders such as vitiligo, lichen planus, seborrheic dermatitis, or contact dermatitis substantially altered the incidence or outcomes of pregnancy in a managed care setting. There was no evidence that the presence of any of the skin diseases substantially altered incidence or clinically recognized outcomes of pregnancy in a managed care setting.

Weatherhead et al. (2007) published a literature survey on the question, whether pregnancy affects psoriasis. Chronic plaque psoriasis improves in a considerable number of patients during pregnancy. This improvement has been associated with the down-regulation of T cell proliferation by high concentrations of progesterone. A deterioration of psoriasis, however, is observed in 10–20% of women during pregnancy. On the other hand, psoriasis

Table 9.4 Dermatoses affected by pregnancy (Kumari et al. 2007)

Diseases	No. of cases	Course
Atopic dermatitis	4	No change
Eczemas	7	Exacerbated
polymorphous light eruption	7	No change
Psoriasis	1	Exacerbated
Acne vulgaris	15	Exacerbated
Vaginal candidosis	17	New onset
Tinea versicolor	11	New onset
Tinea corporis	5	New onset
Herpes labialis	1	New onset
Molluscum contagiosum	1	No change
Verruca vulgaris	2	Exacerbated
Skin tags (Acrohordons)	3	Exacerbated
Melanocytic nevi	2	Exacerbated
Vitiligo	1	New onset
SLE	1	Exacerbated

per se does not affect fertility or rates of miscarriage, birth defects, or premature birth, but some treatment moieties imply potential problems during pregnancy including statements on the safety of antipsoriatic treatment during pregnancy (Table 9.5).

Further knowledge on the relation of autoimmune diseases to pregnancy is limited. Usually, systemic sclerosis does not affect maternal conditions and foetal health during pregnancy (Steen, 2007). The number of pregnancies was not higher in pregnancy cases than in the controls in 210 patients with pemphigus as compared to 205 control patients.

Many women experience some degree of hirsutism on the face, limbs, and back during pregnancy. It resolves postpartum. Pregnant women also may notice mild thickening of scalp hair, due to a prolonged anagen phase. A prolonged telogen phase occurs postpartum, which may cause increased hair shedding (telogen effluvium) for several months (Tunzi and Gray, 2007).

The development of spider telangiectasias (spider nevi) is common, since the peripheral blood vessels are dilated and unstable during pregnancy. Palmar erythema occurs in about two thirds of light-complexioned pregnant women. Saphenous, vulvar, or hemorrhoidal varicosities occur in about 40% women. Vasomotor instability also may cause facial flushing; dermatographism; hot and cold sensations; and marble skin (cutis marmorata). All pregnant women experience some gingival hyperaemia, which may be associated with bleeding (Tunzi and Gray 2007).

60 to 88% of women develop striae during pregnancy (Ghasemi et al. 2007; Osman et al. 2007; Thomas and Liston 2004). Risk factors are: family history of striae in the mother, baseline and delivery body mass index, greatest abdominal and hip girths, newborn weight, height and head circumference (Table 9.6). Influence of family history is strong, Chang et al. (2004) reported an OR of 7.0 (CI 2.7–18.6) for striae, where the mothers had also developed striae in their pregnancies. In addition, 81% of women with striae versus 30.5% without striae reported a history of breast or thigh striae outside the pregnancy.

Table 9.5 Safety of antipsoriatic treatment in pregnancy (Weatherhead et al. 2007)

Safe treatments	Relatively safe treatments (be cautious)	Treatments to be avoided	Treatments with unknown effects	Drug-free interval before conception
Emollients, topical steroids (mild, moderate, or potent), dithranol; ultraviolet B	coal tar products, very potent topical steroids (small quantities); ciclosporin	Topical retinoids, calcipotriol derivatives retinoids, methotrexate, psoralen plus ultraviolet A	Fumaric acid esters; biological agents; hydroxycarbamide	Methotraxte 3 months; retinoids 2 years

Table 9.6 Numeric factors and characteristics of women with and without striae gravidarum (SG) and their newborns. Data shown as median (minimum, maximum, interquartile range) (Ghasemi et al. 2007)

	With SG	Without SG	P-value
Age (year)	23.0 (15.0–36.0)	24.5 (20.0–37.0)	0.29
Height (cm)	160.0 (136.0–178.0)	160.50 (154.0–175.0)	0.63
Baseline BMI (kg m^{-2})	23.8 (16.8–39.5)	22.2 (16.1–26.3)	0.04
Delivery BMI (kg m^{-2})	29.7 (20.6–43.9)	27.5 (24.4–30.8)	0.01
Greatest abdominal girth (cm)	106.0 (73.0–132.0)	100.0 (90.0–127.0)	0.02
Newborn			
Weight (g)	3,225.0 (1,700.0–4,200.0)	3,100.0 (1,750.0–3,300.0)	0.01
Height (cm)	50.0 (43.0–56.0)	49.5 (46.0–53.0)	0.046
Head circumference (cm)	35.0 (29.0–38.0)	34.3 (30.5–36.0)	0.01

9.1.4
Pregnancy and Skin Tumours

Immune Phenomena in Pregnancy. Progesterone is required for implantation and pregnancy maintenance. Progesterone maintains embryo viability, presumably indirectly through its action on uterus. Administration of antiprogestins inhibits implantation and embryo development (Ghosh and Sengupta 1998). Maintenance of the corpus luteum function and its progesterone secretion necessary for decidualization after conception, relies on the influence of hCG, which is produced by the decidua (Alexander et al. 1998).

There is an intense cross-talk between steroid hormones and the immune regulation of endometrium function (Lea and Sandra 2007). Endometrial differentiation, proliferation, cell survival, leukocyte recruitment, apoptosis, and angiogenesis are triggered by sex steroids. Survival factors such as phosphoinositol 3-kinase/protein kinase B, PTEN, NFkappaB, and apoptotic molecules (Fas-FasL, Bcl-2) are regulated by estrogen and progesterone in the endometrium. The steroid hormones are directly active in the expression of chemotactic cytokines (interleukin-8 and monocyte chemotactic protein-1) and on the survival versus apoptosis of resident endometrial cells (stromal, epithelial, and endothelial cells) and non-resident cells (leukocytes) (Kayisli et al. 2004).

The lack of the immune rejection of the embryo and foetus is based on site-specific immunosuppression at the foetal–maternal interface, which allows uninhibited peripheral immune response of the mother (Koch and Platt 2007). CD4(+)CD25(+) Treg cells play essential roles in the induction and maintenance of tolerance. Not only Treg cells but also regulatory NK cells may inhibit maternal T cell or NK cell foetal attack, making the 'Th1/Th2 paradigm of pregnancy' as formulated previously, more complex (Saito et al. 2007). High levels of progesterone during pregnancy contribute to the induction of Th2-type cytokines (Arck et al. 2007). In addition, uterine dendritic cells within the decidua are implicated in pregnancy maintenance (Blois et al. 2007).

Cutaneous Manifestations. A number of common skin tumours iincluding pyogenic granuloma, molluscum fibrosum gravidarum, and skin tags develop more frequently in pregnant than in non-pregnant women (Errickson and Matus 1994) The most common malignancies associated with pregnancy include cervical cancer, breast cancer, melanoma, lymphomas and leukaemia. The incidence of melanoma, which accounts for about 8% of the malignancies, is reported with 2.8 per 1,000 deliveries (Silipo et al. 2006). The question whether the course of melanoma is altered by a pregnancy has often been discussed in literature on the subject. In earlier years, it was a doctrine that a woman who had melanoma should not become pregnant. Many authors suggested that pregnancy increases the risk of developing melanoma and that it has a significantly adverse effect on melanoma disease. In some series, women who were pregnant at the time of diagnosis exhibited an unfavourable survival. More recent studies, however, refuted this suggestion. Also the monitoring of nevi in pregnancy has failed to reveal any reliable changes (Rubegni et al. 2007). In some series multiple previous pregnancies argued for a favourable prognosis and less multiparous women presented more with metastatic disease than nulliparous women. There was no association between enhanced levels of estrogen or progesterone or those of α-MSH in pregnancy (Rampen 1984). Also Grin et al. (1998) stated that the controlled trials available gave no evidence of an influence of pregnancy before, during or after the diagnosis of melanoma on the 5-year survival rates. The same was true for the use of oral contraceptives or hormone replacement therapy after menopause. Again in 2006, a review published by Silipo et al. underlined that there was no significant difference in outcome and survival rate between pregnant and non-pregnant women with melanoma.

9.2
Autoimmune Progesterone Dermatitis

Aetiopathogenesis. Autoimmune progesterone dermatitis (APD) is a rare disease. In 2002, Oskay et al. quoted 10 reports found in literature, but Snyder and Krishnaswamy had in 2003 estimated a number of 50 cases, but not all of them fulfilled all diagnostic criteria. Frequently patients have a history of exogenous progesterone intake (contraceptive pill or progesterone releasing intrauterine device). The aetiopathogenesis of the disease is not very clear; the autoimmune origin not sufficiently proven. Many questions concerning APD are unanswered: Why is the reaction to progesterone expressed primarily at the cutaneous level? Why are direct cutaneous immune fluorescence and intra-dermal skin test reaction to progesterone sometimes negative? Why do eruptions recur during pregnancy whereas others disappear? Why are so many compounds effective in treatment? (Dedecker et al. 2005).

Cutaneous Manifestation. The description of autoimmune progesterone dermatitis comprises a number of dermatologic conditions, including eczema, purpura, erythema multiforme (Fig. 9.5) and Stephen–Johnson syndrome (Fig. 9.6), fixed drug eruption, folliculitis, vesicobullous eruption, and urticaria (Snyder and Krishnaswamy 2003; Baptist and Baldwin 2004; Wintzen et al. 2004; Dedecker et al. 2005; Stranahan et al. 2006).

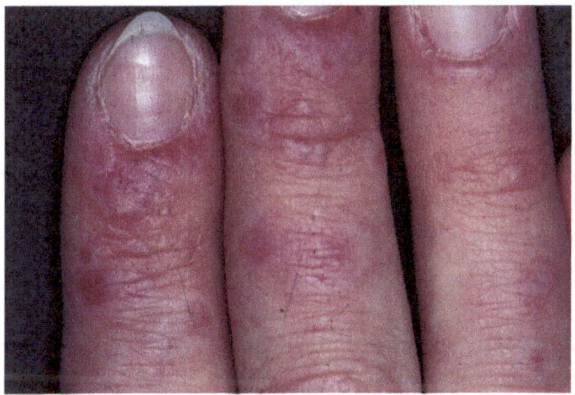

Fig. 9.5 Erythema multiforme as occurring in autoimmune progesterone dermatitis. Lesion begins as a circular red macule, which enlarges centrifugally. While the periphery remains erythematous, the centre becomes cyanotic or purpuric, forming characteristic concentric target lesion

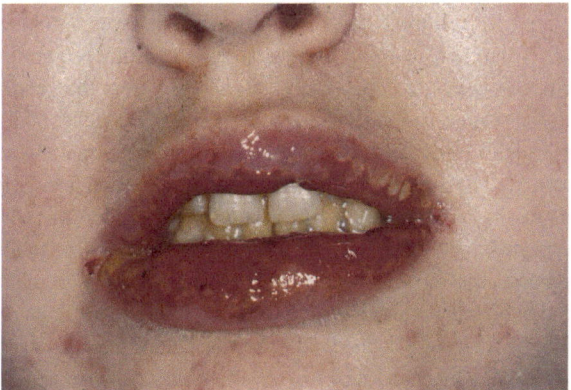

Fig. 9.6 Stephen–Johnson syndrome as occurring in autoimmune progesterone dermatitis. Erythema multiforme maius involves mucous membranes. Lips become erythematous and edematous, secondarily covered by characteristic massive hemorrhagic crusts.Leisons are severely painful, making eating and breathing difficult

Usually, eruptions begin 7 days before menses and resolve 1–3 days thereafter. The spontaneous resolution without residuals is essential for diagnosis. In some cases, mucosal lesions of the oral cavity or colon inducing abdominal pain were associated with skin lesions (Dedecker et al. 2005). In the case reported by Wilkinson et al. (1995) a 31-year-old patient had a history of urticaria occurring every month, beginning mid-cycle and resolving within 3 days of menstruation. She had written a diary to confirm the relationship to the menstrual cycle. The disease had started after she had given birth to a second child and lasted for 6 months until the next pregnancy, during which she remained free of symptoms. The urticaria relapsed following delivery. When taking the history, no changes in diet, cosmetics, or medications as possible causes of allergic reactions could be identified. Serum levels of progesterone, estrogens and gonadotropins were found to be in the normal range. After application of medroxyprogesterone acetate to control endometriosis, she developed severe urticaria for 2 months.

The natural course of APD is variable. The disease can heal spontaneously, and a resolution is observed with menopause. Many patients report a history of application of exogenous gestagens, like the patient of Baptist and Baldwin (2004), who was treated for endometriosis with medroxyprogesterone.

Histopathology. The skin lesions are described as an eosinophilic non-specific vasculitis. They show minimal hyperkeratosis, local parakeratosis, minimal acanthosis and minimal inflammatory infiltrate of mononuclear cells, in part giant cells (Oskay et al. 2002).

Diagnosis. The diagnosis of APD requires recurrent clinical perimenstrual presentations and positive skin test to progesterone. A prick test may be negative, but intracutaneous injection should reveal typical wheals (Baptist and Baldwin 2004; Kakarla and Zurawin 2006; Stranahan et al. 2006; Bemanian et al. 2007). Also serum antibodies reacting with progesterone have been demonstrated. Most case reports described not only antibodies to progesterone of the IgG type, but also high levels of IgE antibodies specific to progesterone, immune complexes and positive basophil degranulation tests (Wilkinson et al. 1995; Dedecker et al. 2005). An invitro IFN-γ-release test, which measures the release of IFN-γ from lymphocytes in culture after challenging with a putative antigen, was found positive. The positive test implies cell mediated immunity with Th1-type cytokine release pattern (Halevy et al. 2002). The sensitization to progesterone does not require previous application of exogenous gestagens. It is not proven in all cases that the sensitizing antigen is indeed progesterone; similar steroids were also suggested (Dedecker et al. 2005).

As the influence of the menstrual cycle on some autoimmune dermatoses and on the reactivity in the prick test is well documented, APD should be differentiated from perimenstrual flares and exacerbations of chronic dermatitis such as acne, psoriasis, lupus erythematosus, atopic dermatitis, lichen planus, and dermatitis herpetiformis (Esteve 1998). In addition, some modulating effects of progesterone on the immune system (stimulation of T-cell rosetting, interleukin production, leukocyte binding to endothelial cells) have also to beconsidered. Since histamine release varies with the menstrual cycle, a pathomechanism of the progesterone related cutaneous lesions outside an antigen–antibody-reaction appears to be possible, originating from hormone-induced alterations of immune functions (Wilkinson et al. 1995).

Treatment. Treatment trials pursued different strategies (Wilkinson et al. 1995; Oskay et al. 2002; Snyder and Krishnaswamy 2003; Dedecker et al. 2005, Kakarla and Zurawin 2006).

Due to the sparseness of the disease, no controlled studies are available. The simplest treatment is that with antihistamines and/or glucocorticoids. Another strategy is the inhibition of endogenous progesterone secretion by ovulation inhibition by estrogens, usually as a formulation of oral contraceptives. Also the depression of ovarial hormone secretion by danazol or GnRH antagonists has been used. These compounds, however, inhibit secretion of ovarian hormones completely and thus induce premature climacterium. Also positive effects of tamoxifen have been described (Cocurroccia et al. 2006). As a definitive treatment, ovariectomy and hysterectomy have been performed in single cases, which is, of course, not adequate in younger women. Immunosuppressive agents such as dapsone, ciclosporine, azathioprine may be effective, but should be avoided because of their possible side effect.

References

Alcalay J, Ingber A, Kafri B, Segal J, Kaufmann H, Hazaz B, Sandbank M. Hormonal evaluation and autoimmune background in pruritic urticarial papules and plaques of pregnancy. Am J Obstet Gynecol. 1988;158(2):417–20.

Alexander H, Zimmermann G, Wolkersdörfer GW, Biesold C, Lehmann M, Einenkel J, Pretzsch G, Baier D. Utero-ovarian interaction in the regulation of reproductive function. Hum Reprod Update. 1998;4(5):550–9.

Ambros-Rudolph CM, Müllegger RR, Vaughan-Jones SA, Kerl H, Black MM. The specific dermatoses of pregnancy revisited and reclassified: results of a retrospective two-center study on 505 pregnant patients. 9a-17. J Am Acad Dermatol. 2006;54(3):395–404.

Arck P, Hansen PJ, Mulac Jericevic B, Piccinni MP, Szekeres-Bartho J. Progesterone during pregnancy: endocrine-immune cross talk in mammalian species and the role of stress. Am J Reprod Immunol. 2007;58(3):268–79.

Aronson IK, Bond S, Fiedler VC, Vomvouras S, Gruber D, Ruiz C. Pruritic urticarial papules and plaques of pregnancy: clinical and immunopathologic observations in 57 patients. J Am Acad Dermatol 1998;39(6): 933–9.

Baptist AP, Baldwin JL. Autoimmune progesterone dermatitis in a patient with endometriosis: case report and review of the literature. Clin Mol Allergy. 2004;2(1):10.

Bemanian MH, Gharagozlou M, Farashahi MH, Nabavi M, Shirkhoda Z. Autoimmune progesterone anaphylaxis. Iran J Allergy Asthma Immunol. 2007;6(2):97–9.

Blois SM, Kammerer U, Alba Soto C, Tometten MC, Shaikly V, Barrientos G, Jurd R, Rukavina D, Thomson AW, Klapp BF, Fernández N, Arck PC. Dendritic cells: key to fetal tolerance? Biol Reprod. 2007;77(4):590–8.

Buccolo LS, Viera AJ. Pruritic urticarial papules and plaques of pregnancy presenting in the postpartum period: a case report. J Reprod Med. 2005;50(1):61–3.

Chang AL, Agredano YZ, Kimball AB. Risk factors associated with striae gravidarum. J Am Acad Dermatol. 2004;51(6):881–5.

Cocuroccia B, Gisondi P, Gubinelli E, Girolomoni G. Autoimmune progesterone dermatitis. Gynecol Endocrinol. 2006;22(1):54–6.

Cohen LM, Capeless EL, Krusinski PA, Maloney ME. Pruritic urticarial papules and plaques of pregnancy and its relationship to maternal-fetal weight gain and twin pregnancy. Arch Dermatol. 1989;125(11):1534–6.

Daniels TE, Quadra-White C. Direct immunofluorescence in oral mucosal disease: a diagnostic analysis of 130 cases. Oral Surg Oral Med Oral Pathol. 1981;51(1): 38–47.

9

Dedecker F, Graesslin O, Quereux C, Gabriel R. Autoimmune progesterone dermatitis: A rare pathology. Eur J Obstet Gynecol Reprod Biol. 2005;123, 121

Elling SV, McKenna P, Powell FC. Pruritic urticarial papules and plaques of pregnancy in twin and triplet pregnancies. J Eur Acad Dermatol Venereol. 2000;14(5):378–81.

Errickson CV, Matus NR. Skin disorders of pregnancy. Am Fam Physician. 1994;49(3):605–10.

Esteve E. Les dermatoses aux oestrogènes et à la progesterone: une nosologie en devenir. Editorial. Ann Dermatol Venereol. 1998;125:484–5.

Ghasemi A, Gorouhi F, Rashighi-Firoozabadi M, Jafarian S, Firooz A. Striae gravidarum: associated factors. J Eur Acad Dermatol Venereol. 2007;21(6):743–6.

Ghosh D, Sengupta J. Recent developments in endocrinology and paracrinology of blastocyst implantation in the primate. Hum Reprod Update. 1998;4(2):153–68.

Grin CM, Driscoll MS, Grant-Kels JM. The relationship of pregnancy, hormones, and melanoma. Semin Cutan Med Surg. 1998;17(3):167–71.

Halevy S, Cohen AD, Lunenfeld E, Grossman N. Autoimmune progesterone dermatitis manifested as erythema annulare centrifugum: Confirmation of progesterone sensitivity by in vitro interferon-gamma release. J Am Acad Dermatol. 2002;47(2):311–3.

Hertl M. (ed). Autoimmune diseases of the skin: pathogenesis, diagnosis, management. 2nd Ed., Springer, New York, 2005

High WA, Hoang MP, Miller MD. Pruritic urticarial papules and plaques of pregnancy with unusual and extensive palmoplantar involvement. Obstet Gynecol. 2005;105(5 Pt 2):1261–4.

Holmes RC, Black MM. The specific dermatoses of pregnancy. J Am Acad Dermatol. 1983 Mar;8(3):405–12.

Jolliffe DS, Sim-Davis D. Cicatricial pemphigoid in a young girl: report of a case. Clin Exp Dermatol. 1977;2(3): 281–4.

Kakarla N, Zurawin RK. A case of autoimmune progesterone dermatitis in an adolescent female. J Pediatr Adolesc Gynecol. 2006;19(2):125–9.

Kayisli UA, Guzeloglu-Kayisli O, Arici A. Endocrine-immune interactions in human endometrium. Ann N Y Acad Sci. 2004;1034:50–63.

Koch CA, Platt JL. T cell recognition and immunity in the fetus and mother. Cell Immunol. 2007;248(1):12–7.

Kumari R, Jaisankar TJ, Thappa DM. A clinical study of skin changes in pregnancy. Indian J Dermatol Venereol Leprol. 2007;73(2):141.

Lakhdar H, Zouhair K, Khadir K, Essari A, Richard A, Seité S, Rougier A. Evaluation of the effectiveness of a broad-spectrum sunscreen in the prevention of chloasma in pregnant women. J Eur Acad Dermatol Venereol. 2007;21(6):738–42.

Laskaris G, Angelopoulos A. Cicatricial pemphigoid: direct and indirect immunofluorescent studies. Oral Surg Oral Med Oral Pathol. 1981;51(1): 48–54.

Lawley TJ, Hertz KC, Wade TR, Ackerman AB, Katz SI. Pruritic urticarial papules and plaques of pregnancy. JAMA. 1979;241(16):1696–9.

Lea RG, Sandra O. Immunoendocrine aspects of endometrial function and implantation. Reproduction. 2007;134(3):389–404.

Matz H, Orion E, Wolf R. Pruritic urticarial papules and plaques of pregnancy: polymorphic eruption of pregnancy (PUPPP). Clin Dermatol. 2006;24(2):105–8.

Muzaffar F, Hussain I, Haroon TS. Physiologic skin changes during pregnancy: a study of 140 cases. Int J Dermatol. 1998;37(6):429–31.

Nilles M, Weyers W, Gründer K. Die PUPPP Dermatose. Hautarzt. 1989;40(9):586–8.

Ohel I, Levy A, Silberstein T, Holcberg G, Sheiner E. Pregnancy outcome of patients with pruritic urticarial papules and plaques of pregnancy. J Matern Fetal Neonatal Med. 2006;19(5):305–8.

Oskay T, Kutluay L, Kaptanoglu A, Karabacak O. Autoimmune progesterone dermatitis. Eur J Dermatol. 2002;12(6):589–91.

Osman H, Rubeiz N, Tamim H, Nassar AH. Risk factors for the development of striae gravidarum. Am J Obstet Gynecol. 2007;196(1):62.e1–5.

Rampen FH. Sex differences in survival from cutaneous melanoma. Int J Dermatol. 1984;23(7): 444–52.

Roger D, Vaillant L, Fignon A, Pierre F, Bacq Y, Brechot JF, Grangeponte MC, Lorette G. Specific pruritic diseases of pregnancy. A prospective study of 3192 pregnant women. Arch Dermatol. 1994;130(6):734–9.

Rubegni P, Sbano P, Burroni M, Cevenini G, Bocchi C, Severi FM, Risulo M, Petraglia F, Dell'Eva G, Fimiani M, Andreassi L. Melanocytic skin lesions and pregnancy: digital dermoscopy analysis. Skin Res Technol. 2007;13(2):143–7.

Saito S, Shiozaki A, Sasaki Y, Nakashima A, Shima T, Ito M. Regulatory T cells and regulatory natural killer (NK) cells play important roles in feto-maternal tolerance. 9: Semin Immunopathol. 2007;29(2):115–22.

Seeger JD, Lanza LL, West WA, Fernandez C, Rivero E. Pregnancy and pregnancy outcome among women with inflammatory skin diseases. Dermatology. 2007;214(1):32–9.

Sheiner E, Ohel I, Levy A, Katz M. Pregnancy outcome in women with pruritus gravidarum. J Reprod Med. 2006;51(5):394–8.

Sherard GB 3rd, Atkinson SM Jr. Focus on primary care: pruritic dermatological conditions in pregnancy. Obstet Gynecol Surv. 2001;56(7):427–32.

Silipo V, De Simone P, Mariani G, Buccini P, Ferrari A, Catricala C. Malignant melanoma and pregnancy. Melanoma Res. 2006;16(6):497–500.

Snyder JL, Krishnaswamy G. Autoimmune progesterone dermatitis and its manifestation as anaphylaxis: a case report and literature review. Ann Allergy Asthma Immunol. 2003;90:469–77.

Steen VD. Pregnancy in scleroderma. Rheum Dis Clin North Am. 2007;33(2):345–58, vii.

Stranahan D, Rausch D, Deng A, Gaspari A. The role of intradermal skin testing and patch testing in the diagnosis of autoimmune progesterone dermatitis. Dermatitis. 2006;17(1):39–42.

Thomas RG, Liston WA. Clinical associations of striae gravidarum. J Obstet Gynaecol. 2004;24(3): 270–1.

Tunzi M, Gray GR. Common Skin Conditions During Pregnancy. Fam Physician. 2007;75:211–8

Uhlin SR. Pruritic urticarial papules and plaques of pregnancy. Involvement in mother and infant. Arch Dermatol. 1981;117(4):238–9.

Vaughan Jones SA, Hern S, Nelson-Piercy C, Seed PT, Black MM. A prospective study of 200 women with dermatoses of pregnancy correlating clinical findings with hormonal and immunopathological profiles. Br J Dermatol. 1999;141(1):71–81.

Weatherhead S, Robson SC, Reynolds NJ. Management of psoriasis in pregnancy. BMJ. 2007;334(7605): 1218–20.

Weiss R, Hull P. Familial occurrence of pruritic urticarial papules and plaques of pregnancy. J Am Acad Dermatol. 1992;26(5 Pt 1):715–7.

Wilkinson SM, Beck MH, Kingston TP. Progesterone-induced urticaria –need it be autoimmune? Br J Dermatol. 1995;133:792–4.

Wintzen M, Goor-van Egmond MB, Noz KC. Autoimmune progesterone dermatitis presenting with purpura and petechiae. Clin Exp Dermatol. 2004;29(3):316.

Zampetti A, Feliciani C, Landi F, Capaldo ML, Rotoli M, Amerio PL. Management and dermoscopy of fast-growing nevi in pregnancy: case report and literature review. J Cutan Med Surg. 2006;10(5):249–52.

Zampino MR, Corazza M, Costantino D, Mollica G, Virgili A. Are melanocytic nevi influenced by pregnancy? A dermoscopic evaluation. Dermatol Surg. 2006;32(12):1497–504.

Zurn A, Celebi CR, Bernard P, Didierjean L, Saurat JH. A prospective immunofluorescence study of 111 cases of pruritic dermatoses of pregnancy: IgM anti-basement membrane zone antibodies as a novel finding. Br J Dermatol. 1992;126(5): 474–8.

Synopsis

Diabetis Mellitus

› Diabetic dermopathy is the most common skin disease in diabetes; it is present in nearly half of diabetic patients older than 50 years. It is caused by diabetic micro-angiopathy, polyneuropathy and infections frequently associated with retinopathy or nephropathy. The typical lesions are flat scars ulcers and bullae mainly at the legs. Fifteen percent of individuals with diabetes develop a foot ulcer during their lifetime- a risk factor for subsequent amputations. Treatment mainly means prevention of ulcers. Correct foot care is mandatory.

› Skin reaction to insulin therapy occur in 5–10% of patients. There are local and systemic allergic reactions including erythema, itching, urticae and infiltrated plaques, urticaria and anaphylactic shock. A special feature is lipoatrophy occurring at the injection sites. Treatment depends on the severity of the phenomena. Frequent change of injection site is advisable. Antihistamines may suppress the itching. In lipatropy, treatment with glucocorticoids has been useful.

› Necrobiosis lipoidica diabeticorum is a slowly progressing, granulomatous disorder of unknown etiology, usually occurring on the pretibial areas. The skin is atrophic and yellowish–brown, enlarged vessels may be seen through the translucent skin. Histopathologically, large areas of necrobiosis in the dermis are seen, surrounded by infiltrates of epithelioid cells, lymphocytes and multinucleate giant cells. A great variety of regimen has been proposed. It appears that NLD is associated with poor glucose control.

› Scleredema adultorum is associated with diabetes mellitus, but association with paraproteinemias and myeloma has also been reported. The skin is tight, thickened and hardened, involving neck, chest, shoulders, and the upper back. The patients report limitation of motion in the joints. Histopathological, the dermis is thickened, the collagen fibres appear to be swollen and separated by wide spaces (dermal fenestration). For treatment, physiotherapy as well as with antibiotics, glucocorticoids, immunosuppressants, and photopheresis were applied. Photochemotherapy appears to be the treatment of choice.

Continued

Walter K. H. Krause, *Cutaneous Manifestations of Endocrine Diseases*,
DOI: 10.1007/978-3-540-88367-8, © Springer-Verlag Berlin Heidelberg 2009

10

> ## Synopsis *Continued*
>
> *Glucagonoma Syndrome*
>
> ❭ Necrolytic migratory erythema as the skin manifestation of glucagonoma
> syndrome is the first symptom of glucagonoma in roughly 79% of patients, its first
> symptoms being macules, bullae and crusted plaques. Later the central part of the
> lesions heals leaving postinflammatory hyperpigmentation, giving the lesions an
> annular appearance. Histopathologically, the epidermis shows clefts in the
> upper spinous cell layer and a diffuse epidermal pallor. Treatment requires surgical
> exstirpation of the underlying tumour. Skin lesions then clear within a week.

10.1   Diabetes Mellitus

10.1.1   Diabetic Dermopathy

Incidence. Patients with insulin dependent diabetes mellitus (IDDM) are susceptible for
various skin diseases. Yosipovitch et al. (1998) studied 238 patients with IDDM and compared the skin lesions to 122 healthy volunteers of comparable age. The most frequent
skin disease in diabetic patients were ichthyosiform skin changes (48%; 6.5% in healthy
persons), scleroderma-like changes (39%; 0% in healthy persons), keratosis pilaris (21%;
9% in healthy persons), and tinea pedis (32%; no data on healthy persons). Scleroderma-
like changes increased significantly with the duration of diabetes. Keratosis pilaris was
associated with the BMI, while the incidence of tinea pedis was associated with age. Of
100 consecutive diabetic outpatients studied by Vijayasingam et al. (1988) 23 had diabetic
dermopathy; 10 of 34 patients using insulin had lipodystrophy, 12 patients had acanthosis
nigricans, and eight patients had xanthelasmata. Romano et al. (1998) found skin diseases
in 276 of 457 diabetic patients. The most frequent skin lesions observed were vitiligo
and psoriasis, followed by xerosis, warts, eczema, mycotic and bacterial infections. The
frequency of skin infections was significantly higher in poorly controlled patients than in
those with good metabolic control. Skin infections were mainly localized at the interdigital
spaces, skin folds and genitalia. Similar figures were described also by Diris et al. (2003)
in 308 diabetic patients and Foss et al. (2005) in 400 diabetic patients. Frequency of skin
lesions was not significantly different between the groups with type I and type II diabetes
except vitiligo, which was significantly more frequent in patients with type I diabetes. The
presence of this autoimmune disorder indicates that autoimmune mechanisms may play a
role also in type I diabetes. The presence of a metabolic syndrome additionally enhances
the risk for ulcerative lesions (Abdul-Ghani et al. 2006).

Aetiopathogenesis. An important cause of skin diseases in diabetes is diabetic microangiopathy, also present in other vascular systems. Microangiopathy is induced by increased
glycosilation end products, oxidative damage, and protein kinase C over activity. Histologically, capillaries and arterioles show thickening of the intima, focal deposits of PAS-positive

material and extravasation of erythrocytes and leukocytes. The metabolism of the vascular walls is altered due to changes of the collagen types and decrease of water binding capacity. The permeation of granulocytes through the vascular wall is inhibited; the phagocytic activity of leukocytes is decreased. Tissue S(HSI)O2 is reduced in the skin of patients with diabetes, and this impairment is accentuated in the presence of neuropathy in the diabetic foot (Greenman et al. 2005). Changes due to microangiopathy are associated with abnormalities of skin perfusion. Capillaries are diminished, which leads to a decrease in perfusion reserve. This is of relevance especially in thermal stimulation. The changes increase with the duration of the disease (Wigington et al. 2004; Ngo et al. 2005).

Diabetic dermopathy appears to be a marker of other vascular complications in diabetes mellitus, such as retinopathy or nephropathy (Vijayasingam et al. 1988; Shemer et al. 1998; Romano et al. 1998; Yosipovitch et al. 1998). Patients suffering from dermopathy are more prone to also suffer from retinopathy or nephropathy than those without dermopathy. The odds ratio for having retinopathy together with dermopathy was estimated as 3.6 (95% CI 1.53–8.44) (Abdollahi et al. 2007)

Further peripheral polyneuropathy, which is a frequent symptom in long-standing diabetes, contributes to skin changes. An increasing intensity of polyneuropathy appears to promote diabetic dermopathy and diabetic ulcer. Patients with diabetic foot ulcer showed a loss of superficial pain sensitivity, perception of pressure and vibration sense. The mean nerve conduction velocities were slower in patients with diabetic dermopathy and diabetic foot ulcer than in patients with onlypolyneuropathy (Kiziltan et al. 2006). Neuropathy is present in over 80% of patients with foot ulcers, promoting ulcer formation by decreasing pain sensation and perception of pressure as well as by causing muscle imbalance.

The third causative factor in diabetic dermopathy is infection. Bacterial infections are mostly caused by *S. aureus*, and also to a lesser extent by enterococcae and *E. coli*. It is not unusual that multiple bacterial species are noted ; in a number of cases no common antibiotic is available. In up to 80% of severe infections anaerobic bacteria are found and may be accompanied by general symptoms ('Diabetic foot flu'). Also there is an increase of incidence of tinea and onychomycosis.

Cutaneous Manifestation. Diabetic dermopathy is the most common skin disease in diabetes; it is present in nearly half of diabetic patients older than 50 years (Wiginton et al. 2004). The symptoms are typical lesions such as multiple, circumscribed, round to oval, red–brownish flat scars, mostly in a pretibial localisation; but flat ulcers in sclerotic skin areas similar to lesions in venous deficiency are also observed (Fig. 10.1). Cutaneous inflammation may also induce bullae (bullosis diabeticorum, Fig. 10.2); Measurement of blood flow demonstrated that lesions do not represent local ischemia, but the scars are a consequence of defective wound healing.

The main focus of skin diseases are the feet (Fig. 10.3). Fifteen percent of individuals with diabetes develop a foot ulcer during their lifetime and 85% of lower extremity amputations are preceded by an ulcer with or without infection. A strong correlation was noted between diabetes-associated foot morbidity and morbid obesity (Pinzur et al. 2005).

In patients with diabetic dermopathy, screening for vascular disease is mandatory. It includes: peripheral pulses, skin temperature, skin thickness, and skin colour. As differential diagnosis, venous insufficiency and arterial occlusive diseases have to be ruled out (Richardson and Kerr 2003).

Fig. 10.1 Diabetic dermopathy. Multiple flat ulcers and scars, mostly in a pretibial localisation

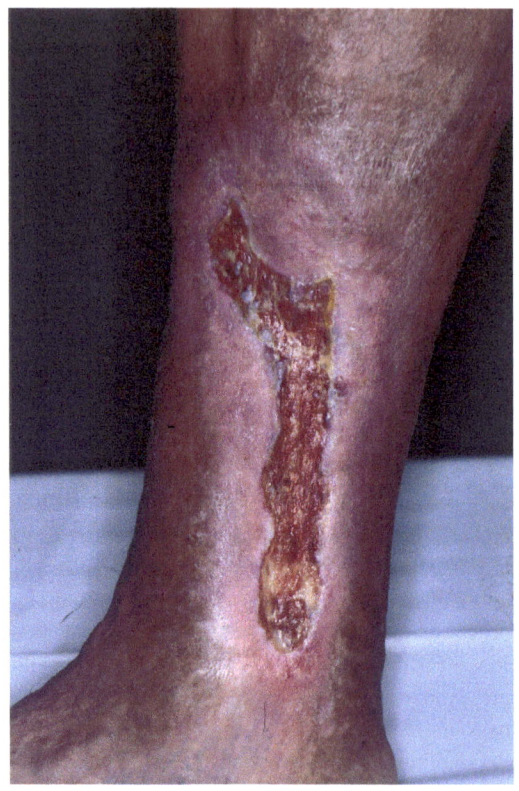

Histopathology. Early lesions present with mild spongiosis of the epidermis and parakeratosis, oedema of the papillary dermis, a mild perivascular infiltrate and extravasated erythrocytes. Figures of neovacularisation of the papillary dermis as well as thickening of the walls of small blood vessels in the dermis and subcutis as well as hemosiderin and siderophages have been found in atrophic lesions.

Treatment. In order to prevent ulcers the rules for foot care in diabetes should be strictly followed (Table 10.1). If foot care education in patients is adequate and skin changes are intensely treated, patients have significantly lower incidence of diseases. Also training of the health personnel significantly improved skin health in the observed diabetics (Brownlee et al. 2003; Frykberg 2003).

Antibacterial treatment is allowed topically only in slight or moderate infections; in all other cases such as cellulitis, lymphangitis, deep ulceration, necrosis, gangrene, osteomyelitis only systemic antibiotics related to bacterial species and sensitivity should be used. Wound debridement is mandatory. A rather new treatment is vacuum therapy. Its use in foot and ankle surgery leads to a quicker wound closure and, in most patients, it helps avoid further surgery (Mendonca et al. 2005)

Foot infections and ulcer are risk factors for subsequent amputations. Osteomyelitis is frequent in diabetic feet; in particular those patients, in whom bone is visible in the ulcer, are jeopardized. An interesting option was short-contact application of topical tretinoin, which

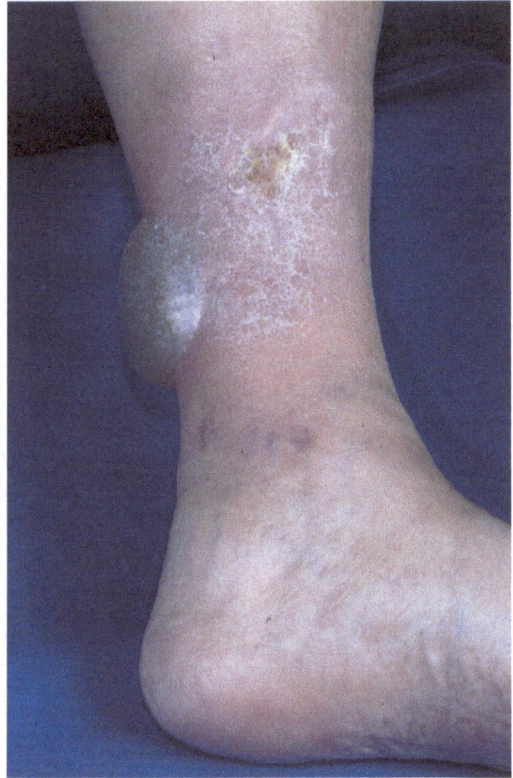

Fig. 10.2 Bullosis diabeticorum. Bullae appearing in the dermopathic skin

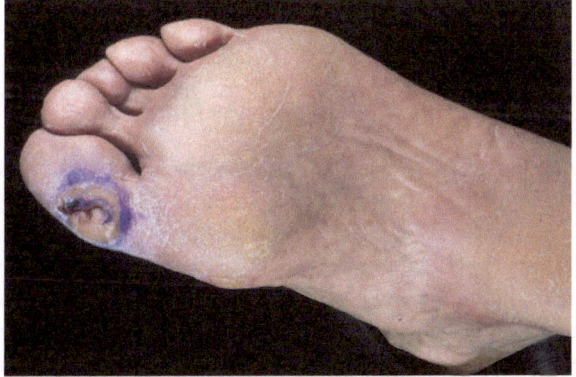

Fig. 10.3 Diabetic foot ulcer. After minimal trauma, chronic wounds develop

Table 10.1 Recommendation for diabetic foot care (From Brownlee et al. 2003; Frykberg 2003)

Disease	Risks	Treatment	Prevention
Pruritus	Scratching, skin defects	Ointments	Avoiding of skin dryness and rifts
Vulnerability	Skin defects, infections	Band aid, warm and comfortable foot wearing	Accurate cleaning, accurate drying after wash, no barefoot walking
Poor wound healing	Ulcers	Avoiding of dents	Accurate rasping of nails, band aid also in small wounds
Tinea (onychomycosis)	Bacterial infections	Antimycotics	Avoid constricting wearing and shoes, avoid cooling
Bacterial infections	Sepsis, osteomyelitis, amputation Cave MRSA, anaerobics	Due to antibiotic testing, topical treatment only in slight to moderate infection. Wound debridement	Avoiding of dents and clavi, no sharp-edged instruments
Diabetic ulcers	Sepsis, osteomyelitis, amputation	Systemic antibiotics, amputation	Avoiding of dents, soft sandals, shoe-lifts

improved the healing of foot ulcers in patients with diabetes. The tretinoin therapy was generally well tolerated, without serious local or systemic adverse effects (Tom et al. 2005).

Dermatomycosis should be treated with oral antimycotics; they are well tolerated, and do not have diabetes-specific side effects. They are far more effective than topical antimycotics particularly in onychomycosis, even if the nail substance is mechanically reduced (Robbins 2003).

10.1.2
Skin Reaction to Insulin Therapy

Incidence. At present, adverse reactions to insulin occur in 5–10% of patients on therapy with insulin. Allergic reactions in general are rare (Linana et al. 1997). Bodtger and Wittrup (2005) observed 22 patients who were suspected to have insulin allergy in 5 years and 6,500 treated patients. However, in nine patients without relevant skin sensitisation the cause was another skin disease, only six patients had allergy to human insulin and three to protamine. In one of the patients, leucocytoclastic vasculitis was demonstrated by histopathological investigation. In the large study ($n = 4,512$) of Fineberg et al. (2003) 2.5% of patients annually were suspected of having insulin allergy, where half of reported events were considered unrelated to insulin therapy. Romano et al. (1998) reported that of 164 patients treated with human insulin, six showed local hypersensitivity reactions and three had generalized urticaria.

Aetiopathogenesis. Allergic reactions to insulin preparations are induced by insulin molecule, altered tertiary structure of insulin, presence of non-insulin protein or pharmaceutical additives, such as protamine sulfate or zinc. Highly purified and biosynthetic insulin preparations are virtually free of protein contaminants. Although insulins of bovine and porcine sources used earlier induced a high rate of allergy – up to 56%, treatment of diabetes using recombinant human insulins also showed a rate of 2.4% of allergic reactions. Insulin antibodies also occur during treatment with human insulin, identical to the original insulin molecule instead of the earlier insulin molecules from antibodies, but to a lesser extent (Wonders et al. 2005). Also purified preparations of human insulin still contain additives and insulin allergies caused by the additives, especially protamine sulfate, still occur (Lee et al. 2002). Protamine-zinc insulin is a retard form of insulin, which is stable in a neutral solution. The most common preparation is NPH (neutral protamine Hagedorn). In some preparations, protamine is replaced by surfen, but this molecule can alsoinduce allergic reactions, at a frequency higher than even protamine. Insulin lispro is an insulin molecule, in which prolin and lysin at position B28 and B29 are interchanged. This alteration does not lead to increased antibody induction (Amon-Herzig-Kellerer 2000).

Closely connected to insulin allergy is lipodystrophy (lipatropy), a rare cutaneous side effect of insulin, occurring at the site of the injections. The atrophy is relevant not only for aesthetic reasons, but also because resorption of injected drugs is reduced in the region. Repeated use of the same injectionsite increases risk of lipoatrophy (Richardson and Kerr 2003; Del Olmo et al. 2008). It was common in the past with the use of animal insulins. It became rare with the introduction of human insulins, but it also occurs with technologically advanced insulin preparations (Arranz et al. 2004; Hussein et al. 2007; Al-Khenaizan et al. 2007; Radermecker et al. 2007). It is closely associated with insulin antibodies in the patients concerned (Raile et al. 2001) and histopathologic examinations of the atrophic tissue gave evidence of an autoimmune activation of macrophages by the complex of insulin (Shimizu et al. 2007). Already Brue et al. (1996) found a dramatic increase of the in vitro production ofTNF-alpha and IL-6 by the macrophages of the patient in presence of insulin in comparison with control subjects. This process required cooperation with other lymphoid cells. Also a local activation of TNF-α plays a role (Ramos and Farias 2006). Altogether, the mechanism of lipatropy is not well understood. A genetic disorder of immune cell function may be the basis (Beltrand et al. 2006).

Cutaneous Manifestations. There are local and systemic allergic reactions to insulin based on specific IgE antibodies. Local reactions may include erythema, itching, urticae and infiltrated plaques in the area of injection. Generalized reactions may present as urticaria and anaphylactic shock.

Diagnosis of allergy to insulin is based on clinical history and cutaneous and serological tests. A definitive skin test method for insulin allergy has yet to be agreed on. Since also the adjuvants of the insulin preparation may induce the allergy, some manufacturers provide a kit including the adjuvants of their preparation in order to facilitate the tests (Wonders et al. 2005).

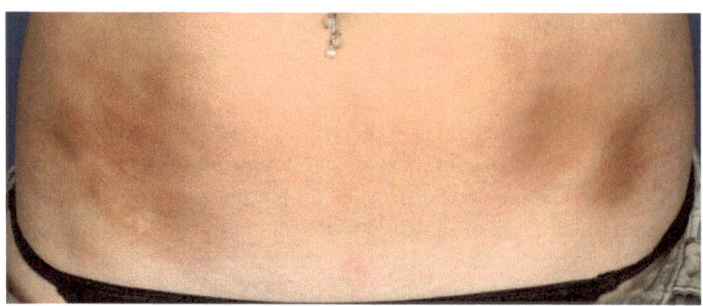

Fig. 10.4 Lipoatrophy caused by insulin injections. Subcutaneous fat is diminished at injection sites

A special feature is lipoatrophy caused by insulin injections. This occurs at the injection sites, occasionally leading to severe deformities of the body shape (Fig. 10.4).

Histopathology. In lipatropy, the volume of the subcutaneous fat and the cell size of the adipocytes are decreased. The adipocytes are separated by a hyalinized or myxoid connective tissue which contains numerous tortuous capillaries. Usually inflammatory changes are absent, but scattered lipophages may be present (Dahl et al. 1996). The changes of the fatty tissue induce figures resembling embryonic fat.

Treatment. Treatment depends on the severity of the phenomena. Local reactions often disappear over time, and also during continued insulin application. Another help may come from the frequent change of injection site. Antihistamines may suppress the itching. If any of the adjuvants causes the allergy, a change of insulin preparation is advisable. Also, if the disease is due to insulin allergy, the first action is the change of insulin preparation. Difficulties are illustrated in the case report of Blanco et al. (1996), who observed a diabetic patient, who exerted severe anaphylactic reaction (self-administered) to neutral protamine Hagedorn human recombinant insulin after subcutaneous injection. He showed local and systemic symptoms, including dyspnoea and hypotension. Positive skin tests and specific IgE to human insulin and protamine were demonstrable. He was treated with human lente insulin and showed tolerance at least for 1 year. Although this patient had real insulin allergy, the protamine allergy was responsible for the disease. Another possibility is the administration of insulin via a subcutaneous infusion using a pump. In severe diseases, a, intravenous insulin application or continuous intraperitoneal insulin unfusion may be applied. Desensitization therapy was also investigated in different regimen (Yokoyama et al. 2003; Castera et al. 2005; Wonders et al. 2005).

In lipatropy, treatment with glucocorticoids has been found to be useful (Ramos and Farias 2006). Lopez et al. (2008) inaugurated the treatment with chromolyn to inhibit insulin-induced lipatropy. They demonstrated a reduction of mast cells at the site of the disease histologically. The likelihood of lipoatrophy can be reduced by regular rotation of injection sites but once developed, practical benefits may be obtained by insulin injection into the edge of the area, co-administration of dexamethasone with insulin, or changing the mode of insulin delivery (Richardson and Kerr 2003).

10.1.3
Necrobiosis Lipoidica Diabeticorum

Aetiopathogenesis. The aetiopathogenesis of necrobiosis lipoidica diabeticorum (NLD) is unknown. Immune pathologic mechanisms are considered to play a role (Wee and Possick 2004). An association to traumata is likely, since it manifests nearly exclusively in the pretibial area and new lesions of NLD may be observed as a Koebner phenomenon. It occurs also in non-diabetic patients.

Cutaneous Manifestation. NLD is a slowly progressing, granulomatous disorder, usually occurring on the pretibial areas. The lesions begin as dark red, elevated nodules with irregular borders. Later, the skin becomes atrophic. The lesion becomes yellowish–brown, only the margin maintains the red colour. (Fig. 10.5). Epidermis is thin and shows minor scaling. Enlarged vessels may be seen through the translucent skin (Fig. 10.6). Subjective sensations are not reported. Tokura et al. (2003) reported on a case with NLD on the glans

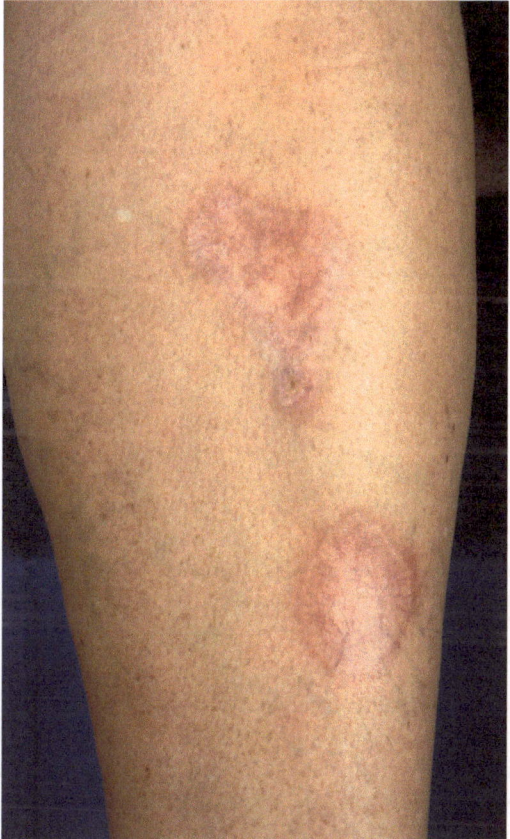

Fig. 10.5 Necrobiosis lipoidica. Lesions begin as dark red, elevated nodules with irregular borders. Later, the skin becomes atrophic. Lesion becomes yellowish–brown, only the margin maintains the red colour

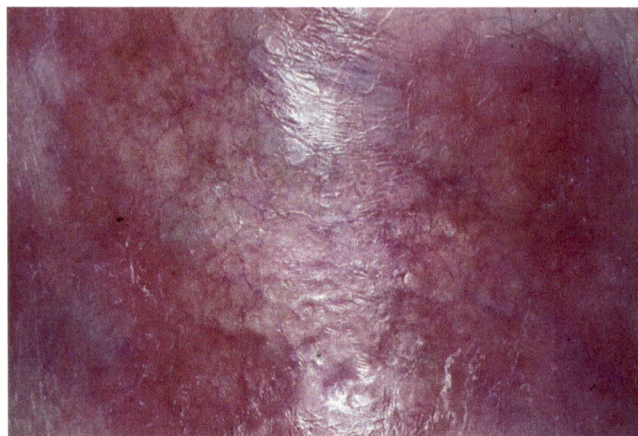

Fig. 10.6 Necrobiosis lipoidica. Atrophic skin with translucent, dilated blood vessels and fatty tissue

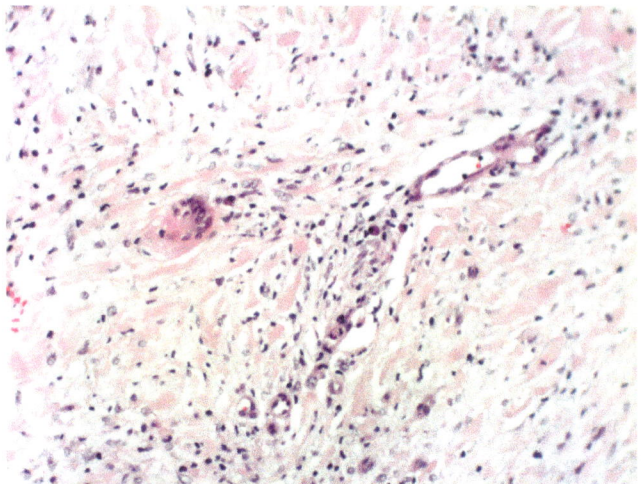

Fig. 10.7 Necrobiosis lipoidica, histopathology. Below an unaltered epidermis, large areas of necrobiosis are visible. They are surrounded by infiltrates of epithelioid, palisading histiocytes, lymphocytes and occasional multinucleate giant cells; plasma cells are usual constituents

penis, presenting as an ulcerative balanitis. Histopathologically the typical palisading granulomas were demonstrable. Lesions of NLD ulcerate in up to 25% patients and this fact has to be considered in the differential diagnosis of leg ulcers. Accompanying diabetic sensory neuropathy may be present. Also, the development of spinal cell carcinoma of the skin within the lesions of NLD was observed (Gudi et al. 2000 McIntosh et al. 2005).

Histopathology. Epidermal lesions may vary between acanthosis, atrophy and hyperkeratosis or an unchanged epidermis (Fig. 10.7). Necrobiosis are present in the mid and lower dermis large areas of. These are surrounded by infiltrates of epithelioid, palisading histiocytes, lymphocytes and occasional multinucleate giant cells, plasma cells are usual

Table 10.2 Reported treatments for necrobiosis lipoidica diabeticorum (Nguyen et al. 2002)

Topical and intralesional glucocorticoids
Systemic corticosteroids
Nicotinamide
Pentoxifylline
Acetylsalicylic acid
Oral ticlopidine
Topical tretinoin
Topical bovine collagen
Hyperbaric oxygen
Porcine dressings, split-thickness skin grafts, pressure garment

constituents. Occasionally eosinophils may also be present. Dermal fibrosis may be seen among the necrobiotic granulomas. A loss of elastic tissue in the necrobiotic areas can be demonstrated by stains for elastin. Further lipid droplets visualized by Sudan stain appear frequently, while cholesterol clefts are a rare feature (Gebauer and Armstrong 1993; De la Torre et al. 1999). Vascular changes appear as endothelial swelling of vessel walls with a lymphocytic vasculitis and perivasculitis. Alteration of the septa of the subcutaneous fat has also been noted.

Treatment. No adequate treatment is known. Table 10.2 lists a number of treatment procedures which were proposed in various reports on the subject (Nguyen et al. 2002). The proposals mainly relate to case reports or small series, a controlled study is reported only for aspirin; the treatment failed to improve the disease. It appears that NLD is associated with poor glucose control; tighter control might improve or prevent this disorder (Cohen et al. 1996). Heavily depressed scars often remain after healing. In recent years, more case reports and small, but uncontrolled studies on the treatment of NLD were published including fumaric esters (Kreuter et al. 2005), ciclosporin (Aslan et al. 2007), anti-TNF α-antibodies (Alexis and Strober 2005), and pioglitazone, an oral antidiabetic drug (Boyd 2007). Topical tacrolimus, which is broadly used in inflammatory skin diseases, was ineffective (Rallis et al. 2007).

10.1.4
Scleredema Adultorum

Aetiopathogenesis. In 1902, Buschke suggested the term 'scleredema adultorum' to distinguish this entity from scleredema neonatorum. There are different types of scleredema adultorum (Table 10.3). 29% of patients in the study of Beers et al. (2006) were 0 to 10 years of age, 22% were 10–20 years, and 48% were older than 20 years. About 400 cases were described in the literature up to now. Most frequently, it was associated with diabetes mellitus (up to 15% of the diabetics in a study), but also cases associated with paraproteinemias and myeloma, with insulinoma, with rheumatoid arthritis and Sjögren's snydrom, and hyperparathyreoidism were reported (Jacob et al. 2002).

Table 10.3 Types of Scleredema adultorum (from Beers et al. 2006)

Type	Patient's ratio		
Type 1	55%	Preceding febrile illness, usually complete spontaneous resolution in months to 2 years.	Classic type described by Buschke
Type 2	25%	No preceding febrile illness, slowly progressive, non-resolving course, risk of developing paraproteinaemias including multiple myeloma.	At younger age hypergamma-globulinaemia is less frequently than in older persons
Type 3	20%	No preceding febrile illness, slowly progressive, non-resolving course	Associated with diabetes mellitus

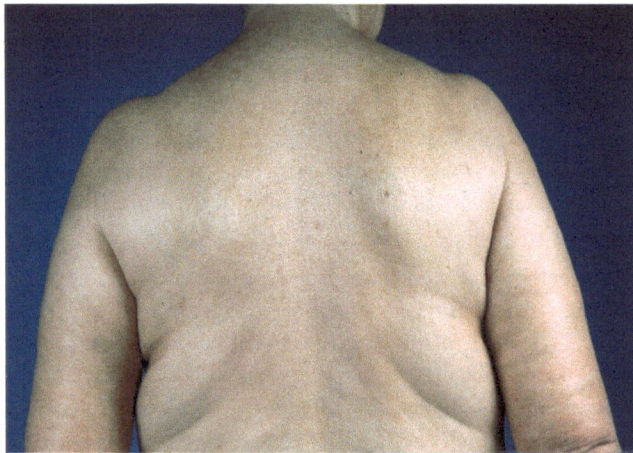

Fig. 10.8 Scleredema adultorum. Lesions involve neck, chest, shoulders, and the upper back, and the disease may progress to the face and to the proximal arms. The patients report limitation of range of motion in the torso, shoulders, and neck

Cutaneuous Manifestations. In scleredema, the skin shows tightness, thickening, and hardening, evolving within months or years. Lesions are seen in the neck, chest, shoulders, and the upper back, and the disease may progress to the face and to the proximal arms (Fig. 10.8). Patients report limitation of range of motion in the torso, shoulders, and neck as well as a decreased oral aperture and difficulty swallowing (Haustein 2005; Beers et al. 2006).

Parmar et al. (2000) reported on a case of an 8-year-old boy where thickening of the skin appeared first in the face, and within ten days it spread over neck, trunk, and arms. 4 weeks earlier , he had suffered from chicken pox. The skin was waxy, with non-pitting swelling, and was not pinchable. The skin folds were obliterated, complete mouth opening was not possible. Within the next 2 weeks, the thickening resolved spontaneously.

Lamba et al. (2005) observed a 65-year-old diabetic man who developed a velvety, hyperpigmented, papillomatous plaque located centrally in diffuse 'wooden' indurate plaque involving the upper midback. The lesion appeared as acanthosis nigricans in a plaque of scleredema. Histologic examination of a skin biopsy revealed epidermal papillomatosis with thickening of the dermis. Since both the skin disorders may occur in diabetes mellitus, the coincidence as observed is not unlikely.

Histopathology. Epidermis is usually not involved. The dermis may be up to four times thicker than normal. The collagen fibres appear to be swollen and separated by wide spaces (dermal fenestration); small amounts of mucin are localized that can be stained by alcian or toluidine blue or colloidal iron. Within the subcutaneous tissue fat is replaced by coarse collagen fibres, thus the eccrine glands appear to be located in the mid-dermis, being tightly enclosed by collagen bundles. The number of fibroblasts is normal or slightly decreased. Inflammation is usuallysmall, the mast cell number may be increased (Truhan and Roenigk 1986). No immune globulin deposits are present (Venencie et al. 1984; McFadden et al. 1987). As differential diagnoses, scleromyxoedema and morphea have to be considered. In scleromyxoedema, there is marked proliferation of fibroblasts and deposits of mucin are usually more prominent. In morphea deep inflammatory infiltrates can be present while the thickened collagen bundles appear hyalinized and paler in HE staining.

The involvement of other organs (heart, bone, jounts, liver, spleen, eye, bone marrow, nerves) in the mucopolysaccharide deposition has been described.

Treatment. No standard treatment exists. Uncontrolled studies report on a treatment by physiotherapy as well as with antibiotics, glucocorticoids, immunosuppressants, photopheresis, and photochemotherapy (Beers et al. 2006). The latter appears to be the treatment of choice (Tuchinda et al. 2006), even if topical UVA1 irradiation needed 35–62 applications in 2–3 months for improvement (Eberlein-König et al. 2005). The condition should not be neglected as spontaneous remission is frequent (Haustein 2005). In the study of Bowen et al. (2003) the underlying hypergammaglobulinaemia was sufficiently treated with electron beam, and improvement of scleredema was noted. As a result of this treatment, shoulder abduction improved in angle from 90 to 180°, percentage of subjective improvement of motion from baseline ranged from 25 to 80%, and the ease of breathing from 33 to 29%.

10.2
Glucagonoma Syndrome

Aetiopathogenesis. Glucagonoma syndrome, which may appear as an isolated disease or as part of multiple endocrine neoplasia (van Beek et al. 2004) is a very rare disorder with an estimated incidence of one in 20 million. The rate of malignancy is high, estimations range from 57 to 100%. The 5-year survival is less than 50% (Kovacs et al. 2006).

The skin manifestation of glucagonoma syndrome necrolytic migratory erythema (NME). NME appears to be a direct consequence of enhanced glucagon levels in serum. It disappears usually within few days after surgical removal of the glucagonoma, parallel to decreasing glucagon levels. The assumption is further supported by the observation of Mullans and Cohen (1998): A patient developed NME after treatment of hypoglycemia induced by an insulin-like growth factor II-secreting haemangiopericytoma with glucagon. Case and Vassilopoulou (2003) reported similar observations: if glucagon is administered as a continuous infusion as an effective treatment of tumour-induced hypoglycemia. the development of NME was observed as a side effect in three cases.

The analysis of the physiological function of glucagon suggests that NME is a true deficiency dermatosis. Hypovitaminosis of B vitamins (Riboflavin, Niacin, Pyroxidine, biotin, and cyanocobalamine) include similar skin lesions. Enhanced protein breakdown leads to deficiency of essential amino acid and essential fatty acids, which may result in deficiency of nerval and vascular active compounds (dopamine, epinephrine, thyroxine, tri-iodothyronine and serotonin). All this may contribute in a complex way to the glucagonoma syndrome. Metabolic alterations may depend on duration and degree of hyperglucagonaemia and (pre-existing) nutritional status of the patient. (Tierney and Badger 2004; van Beek et al. 2004). However, results of in-vitro studies of the skin supporting the hypothesis are not available.

An alternative hypothesis of the pathogenesis of NME is that glucagon induces elevated levels of inflammatory mediators, which in turn i induce epidermal necrolysis. There are, however, no experimental trials which support this suggestion. Immune mechanisms were never taken in consideration in the pathogenesis of NME.

Some authors speculated that the glucagonoma might additionally secrete peptides other than glucagon, which are responsible for the induction of NME (Rappersberger et al. 1987; van Beek et al. 2004). Further, pancreatic polypeptide is very often co-secreted in glucagonomas. High levels of this peptide may potentiate the catabolic effects of glucagon. Kasper and McMurry (1991), on the other hand, suggested that hypergluconaemia is not an essential condition in NME, since they observed a patient who had NME with diabetes and hepatic failure in absence of glucagonoma. In conclusion, the aetiology of NME expects further clarification.

NME was also described outside the glucagonoma syndrome, i.e. without glucagonoma (pseudoglucanoma syndrome). An association with intestinal mal-absorption disorders, liver cirrhosis or hepatitis, inflammatory bowel disease, pancreatitis and malignancies other than pancreatic was described (Tierney and Badger 2004; Marinkovich et al. 1995). A worsening was observed with deterioration of the cirrhosis. A case report (85-year-male) of Technau et al. (2005) described the occurrence of NME in a patient with myelodysplasia. In these patients glucagon levels are also elevated, but not as excessively as in the glucagonoma syndrome. Thus a similar pathogenic origin of skin lesions in both pseudoglucagonoma and glucagonoma syndromes was suggested. The hypotheses include a direct action of glucagons in the skin, glucagons induction of inflammatory mediators, and presence of substance(s) secreted from the pancreatic tumour in addition to glucagons.

Cutaneous Manifestations. NME in association with glucagonoma was first described by Becker et al. in 1942 in a woman with an alpha-cell tumour of the pancreas who had elevated serum glucagon levels and significant hypoaminoacidemia. Since that time, more than 200 cases of the disease were described in the literature (Tierney and Badger 2004). The term 'necrolytic migratory erythema' was first used by Mallinson et al. (1974).

NME is the first symptom of glucagonoma in roughly 79% of patients (van Beek et al. 2004). Wermers et al. (1996) analysed 139 patients with hyperglucagonemia. 21 (11 male, 10 female; age 28–73 year) fulfilled three conditions of the glucagonoma syndrome:

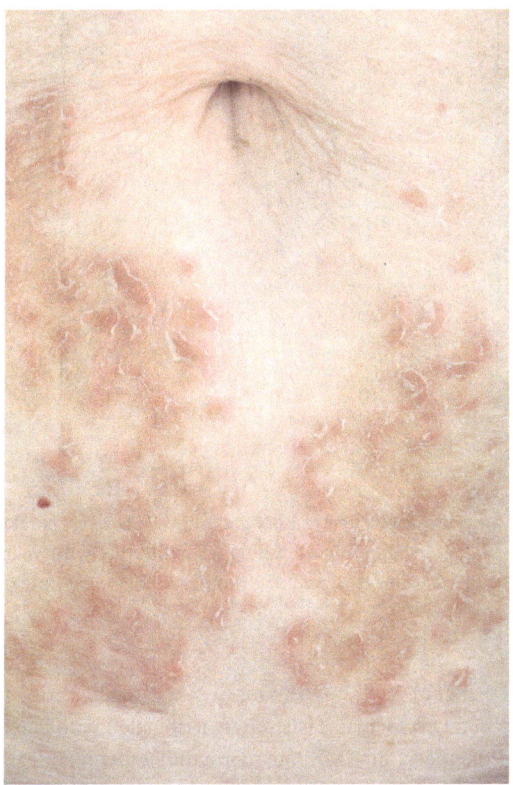

Fig. 10.9 Necrolytic migratory erythema. Lesions show macules, flaccid bullae and crusted plaques occurring mainly at friction sites. Within a few days central part of the lesions heals with postinflammatory hyperpigmentation, giving an annular appearance

had high glucagons levels (>120 pg ml^{-1}), islet cell tumour, and an NME. None of the 21 included subjects had evidence of a secondary cause of hyperglucagonemia. In 14 of the NME was the leading symptom, but in 15 of them it was weight loss, in eight of them diabetes. NME alone was present in five patients.

NME firstly presents with skin lesions occurring in a cyclic pattern: macules, central formation of flaccid bullae and crusted plaques occurring mainly at friction sites. Usually after 1–2 weeks, the central part of the lesions heals leaving post inflammatory hyperpigmentation, giving the lesions an annular appearance. The erythematous periphery thus becomes encrusted. Lesions extend centrifugally, resulting in a serpiginous pattern and become confluent (Fig. 10.9).The main sites are perineum, buttocks, groin, lower abdomen, and lower extremities. In some patients, similar lesions occur at oral (cheilitis and glossitis), genital, and perianal sites (Tierney and Badger 2004; van Beek et al. 2004; Kovacs et al. 2006). In rare cases, the first clues of NME were nail abnormalities brittle nails, onychoschisis (Chao and Lee 2002). Skin lesions and general symptoms such as diabetes mellitus, glossitis, anemia, and weight loss may precede the diagnosis of glucagonoma 1–6 years (Edney et al. 1990). Typically, the lesions of NME cleared after resection of the

10

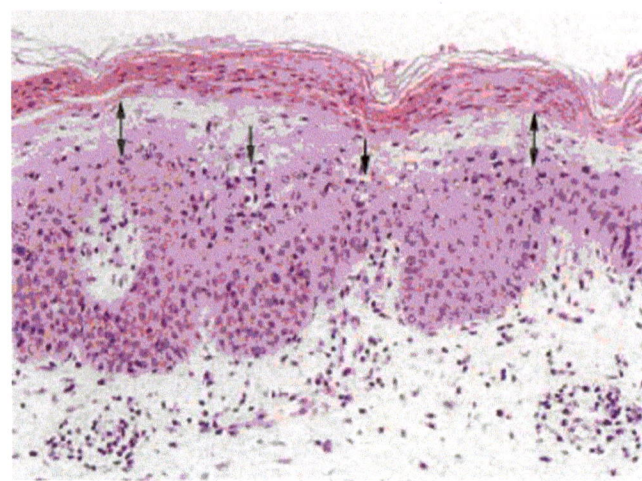

Fig. 10.10 Necrolytic migratory erythema, histopathology. There is parakeratosis, loss of the granular layer, necrosis, and separation of the upper epidermis with vacuolization of the keratinocytes, dyskeratotic keratinocytes, and neutrophils in the upper epidermis (from van Beek et al. 2004, with permission)

glucagonoma (El Rassi et al. 1998). A variant of NME was described by van Beek et al. (2004) as necrolytic acral erythema; it is strongly associated with hepatitis C.

As a differential diagnosis of NME, acrodermatitis enteropathica, pellagra, psoriasis, seborrhoic or contact eczema, pemphigus, essential fatty acid deficiency, annular chronic lupus erythematosus, drug reactions have to be considered (Kovacs et al. 2006; Tierney and Badger 2004).

Acrodermatitis enteropathica is the consequence of zinc deficiency result. It occurs usually in childhood, but is rare in adulthood. It comprises stomatitis, photophobia, nail dystrophyand hair shaft abnormalities. Pellagra develops as a consequence of inadequate amounts of niacin (nicotinic acid) in the tissues. It occurs also as a consequence of carcinoid syndrome, where tumour cells divert tryptophan metabolism toward serotonin and away from nicotinic acid. Also in Hartnup disease, which includes a congenital defect in tryptophan absorption and transfer, a burning erythema in sun-exposed areas with sharply demarcated lesions occurs. (van Beek et al. 2004).

Histopathology. For exact diagnosis, biopsies have to be taken from the edge of an early lesion (Fig. 10.10). The epidermis shows hyperkeratosis, confluent parakeratosis,, akanthotis and clefts in the upper spinous and the granular cell layer. There is a diffuse epidermal pallor, a loss of normal basophilia and hypogranulosis, and clear cells with empty balloon-like or hazy cytoplasm are visible (Long et al. 1993; Tanner et al. 1994; Tierney and Badger 2004). Subcorneal pustulation (Kheir et al. 1986) may be present, sometimes with a polymorph neutrophilic infiltrate. A mild lymphocytic, pervisacular infiltrate in the upper dermis is frequently observed. Using immune histology, apoptotic keratinocytes staining positive with immune globulins, fibrinogen, and C3 are found (Perniciaro et al. 1998). In singular studies, suprabasal acantholysis and isolation of keratinocytes and a reduction of desmosomes without acantholysis have been described (Long et al. 1993). Other rare findings include suppurative folliculitis (Hunt et al. 1991; Kheir et al. 1986; Kovacs et al. 2006), accompanying candidosis (Katz et al. 1979) and focal dyskeratosis (Hunt et al. 1991)which are clues to early diagnosis.

By electron microscopy, the intercellular spaces in the epidermis are found to be enlarged in all layers. The keratinocytes are filled with numerous vesicles, and several structures are lost. The dyskeratotic cells, which are present predominantly in the granular layer, contain fewer desmosomes, their nuclei are pycnotic and only few mitochondria are observed. The basal lamina is unchanged.

With respect to aetiopathogenetic considerations, van Beek et al. (2004) indicated that the histolopathologic appearance of NME is very similar to the biopsy findings in other deficiency states like pellagra, zinc deficiency, and necrolytic acral erythema. Already Franchimont et al. (1982) have observed extensive angioplasia in NME, resembling recalcitrant psoriasis (Johnson et al. 2003). This was confirmed as a common observation by later authors (Kheir et al. 1986).

Treatment. The treatment of NME in glucagonoma syndrome requires the surgical extirpation of the underlying tumour. Skin lesions then clear within 1 week; a recurrence is indicative of a tumour relapse (Smith et al. 1996). No further treatment of cutaneous changes is necessary. Other therapeutic trials were performed using somatostatin (Elsborg and Glenthoj 1985) and octretoide (Camisa 1989). Intermittent infusions of amino acids and fatty acids over 1 year resolved NME in two cases, after a treatment with octretoide had failed or even although the glucagonoma itself remained unchanged (Bewley et al. 1996; Alexander et al. 2002).

Descriptions on the treatment of pseudoglucagonoma syndrome are rare. In the case of Ossowski and Baum (1995), trials with tetracyclin and acitetretin as well as the topical application of triamcinolone remained without success. The lesions cleared, however, within a few days after administration of dapsone 100 mg per day. In the report of Tanner et al. (1994), abstinence from alcohol, controlled nutrition and external wound care cleared the lesions within 10 days.

References

Abdollahi A, Daneshpazhooh M, Amirchaghmaghi E, Sheikhi S, Eshrati B, Bastanhagh. Dermopathy and retinopathy in diabetes: is there an association? Dermatology. 2007;214(2):133–6.

Abdul-Ghani M, Nawaf G, Nawaf F, Itzhak B, Minuchin O, Vardi P. Increased prevalence of microvascular complications in type 2 diabetes patients with the metabolic syndrome. Israel Med Assoc J. 2006;8(6):378–82.

Alexander EK, Robinson M, Staniec M, Dluhy RG. Peripheral amino acid and fatty acid infusion for the treatment of necrolytic migratory erythema in the glucagonoma syndrome. Clin Endocrinol (Oxf). 2002;57(6):827–31.

Alexis AF, Strober BE. Off-label dermatologic uses of anti-TNF-a therapies. J Cutan Med Surg. 2005;9(6):296–302.

Al-Khenaizan S, Al Thubaiti M, Al Alwan I. Lispro insulin-induced lipoatrophy: a new case. Pediatr Diabetes. 2007;8(6):393–6.

Amon-Herzig-Kellerer. Antidiabetica. Wissenschaftliche Verlagsgesellschaft, Stuttgart 2000.

Arranz A, Andia V, López-Guzmán A. A case of lipoatrophy with Lispro insulin without insulin pump therapy. Diabetes Care. 2004;27(2):625–6.

Aslan E, Körber A, Grabbe S, Dissemond J. Erfolgreiche Therapie einer exulzerierten Necrobiosis lipoidica non diabeticorum mit Ciclosporin. Hautarzt. 2007;58(8):684–8.

Beers WH, Ince A, Moore TL. Scleredema adultorum of Buschke: a case report and review of the literature. Semin Arthritis Rheum. 2006;35(6):355–9.

Beltrand J, Guilmin-Crepon S, Castanet M, Peuchmaur M, Czernichow P, Levy-Marchal C. Insulin allergy and extensive lipoatrophy in child with type 1 diabetes. Horm Res. 2006;65(5):253–60.

Bewley AP, Ross JS, Bunker CB, Staughton RC. Successful treatment of a patient with octreotide-resistant necrolytic migratory erythema. Br J Dermatol. 1996;134(6):1101–4.

Blanco C, Castillo R, Quiralte J, Delgado J, Garcia I, de Pablos P, Carrillo T. Anaphylaxis to subcutaneous neutral protamine Hagedorn insulin with simultaneous sensitization to protamine and insulin. Allergy. 1996;51(6):421–4.

Bodtger U, Wittrup M. A rational clinical approach to suspected insulin allergy: status after five years and 22 cases. Diabet Med. 2005;22(1):102–6.

Bowen AR, Smith L, Zone JJ. Scleredema adultorum of Buschke treated with radiation. Arch Dermatol. 2003;139(6):780–4.

Boyd AS. Treatment of necrobiosis lipoidica with pioglitazone. J Am Acad Dermatol. 2007;57 (5 Suppl):S120–1.

Brownlee M, Aiello LP, Friedman E, Vinik AI, Nesto RW, Boulton JM. Complications of diabetes mellitus, pp 1509–84. In: Williams Textbook of Endocrinology, 10th Edition, Eds: Larsen PR, Kronenberg HM, Melmed S, Polonsky KS, Saunders, Philadelphia, 2003

Camisa C. Somatostatin and a long-acting analogue, octreotide acetate. Relevance to dermatology. Arch Dermatol. 1989;125(3):407–12.

Case CC, Vassilopoulou-Sellin R. Reproduction of features of the glucagonoma syndrome with continuous intravenous glucagon infusion as therapy for tumor-induced hypoglycemia. Endocr Pract. 2003;9(1):22–5.

Castera V, Dutour-Meyer A, Koeppel M, Petitjean C, Darmon P. Systemic allergy to human insulin and its rapid and long acting analogs:successful treatment by continuous subcutaneous insulin lispro infusion. Diabet Metab. 2005;31(4 Pt 1):391–400.

Chao SC, Lee JY. Brittle nails and dyspareunia as first clues to recurrences of malignant glucagonoma. Br J Dermatol. 2002;146(6):1071–4.

Cohen O, Yaniv R, Karasik A, Trau H. Necrobiosis lipoidica and diabetic control revisited. Med Hypotheses. 1996;46(4):348–50.

Dahl PR, Zalla MJ, Winkelmann RK. Localized involutional lipoatrophy: a clinicopathologic study of 16 patients. J Am Acad Dermatol. 1996;35(4):523–8.

De la Torre C, Losada A, Cruces MJ. Necrobiosis lipoidica: a case with prominent cholesterol clefting and transepithelial elimination. Am J Dermatopathol. 1999;21(6):575–7.

Del Olmo MI, Campos V, Abellán P, Merino-Torres JF, Piñón F. A case of lipoatrophy with insulin detemir. Diabetes Res Clin Pract. 2008;80(1):e20–1.

Diris N, Colomb M, Leymarie F, Durlach V, Caron J, Bernard P. Dermatoses non infectieuses au cours du diabète sucré: étude prospective de 308 malades. Ann Dermatol Venereol. 2003;130(11): 1009–14.

Eberlein-Konig B, Vogel M, Katzer K, Hein R, Kohn FM, Ring J, Abeck D. Successful UVA1 phototherapy in a patient with scleredema adultorum. J Eur Acad Dermatol Venereol. 2005;19(2):203–4.

Edney JA, Hofmann S, Thompson JS, Kessinger A. Glucagonoma syndrome is an underdiagnosed clinical entity. Am J Surg. 1990;160(6):625–8.

El Rassi Z, Partensky C, Valette PJ, Berger F, Chayvialle JA. Necrolytic migratory erythema, first symptom of a malignant glucagonoma: treatment by long-acting somatostatin and surgical resection. Report of three cases. Eur J Surg Oncol. 1998;24(6):562–7.

Elsborg L, Glenthoj A. Effect of somatostatin in necrolytic migratory erythema of glucagonoma. Acta Med Scand. 1985;218(2):245–9.

Fineberg SE, Huang J, Brunelle R, Gulliya KS, Anderson JH Jr. Effect of long-term exposure to insulin lispro on the induction of antibody response in patients with type 1 or type 2 diabetes. Diabetes Care. 2003;26:89–96.

Foss NT, Polon DP, Takada MH, Foss-Freitas MC, Foss MC. Skin lesions in diabetic patients. Rev Saude Publica. 2005;39(4):677–82.

Franchimont C, Pierard GE, Luyckx AS, Gerard J, Lapiere CM. Angioplastic necrolytic migratory erythema. Unique association of necrolytic migratory erythema, extensive angioplasia, and high molecular weight glucagon-like polypeptide. Am J Dermatopathol. 1982;4(6):485–95.

Frykberg RG. An evidence-based approach to diabetic foot infections. Am J Surg. 2003;186(5A): 44S–54S

Gebauer K, Armstrong M. Koebner phenomenon with necrobiosis lipoidica diabeticorum. Int J Dermatol. 1993;32(12):895–6.

Greenman RL, Panasyuk S, Wang X, Lyons TE, Dinh T, Longoria L, Giurini JM, Freeman J, Khaodhiar L, Veves A. Early changes in the skin microcirculation and muscle metabolism of the diabetic foot. Lancet. 2005;366(9498):1711–7.

Gudi VS, Campbell S, Gould DJ, Marshall R. Squamous cell carcinoma in an area of necrobiosis lipoidica diabeticorum: a case report. Clin Exp Dermatol. 2000;25(8):597–9.

Haustein UF. Scleroderma and pseudo-scleroderma: uncommon presentations. Clin Dermatol. 2005;23(5):480–90.

Hunt SJ, Narus VT, Abell E. Necrolytic migratory erythema: dyskeratotic dermatitis, a clue to early diagnosis. J Am Acad Dermatol. 1991;24(3):473–7.

Hussein SF, Siddique H, Coates P, Green J. Lipoatrophy is a thing of the past, or is it? Diabet Med. 2007;24(12):1470–2.

Jacob N, Gleichmann U, Stadler R. Sclerödema adultorum Buschke bei secundärem Hyperparathyroidismus. Hautarzt. 2002;53(2):121–5.

Johnson SM, Smoller BR, Lamps LW, Horn TD. Necrolytic migratory erythema as the only presenting sign of a glucagonoma. J Am Acad Dermatol. 2003;49(2):325–8.

Kasper CS, McMurry K. Necrolytic migratory erythema without glucagonoma versus canine superficial necrolytic dermatitis: is hepatic impairment a clue to pathogenesis? J Am Acad Dermatol. 1991;25(3):534–41.

Katz R, Fischmann AB, Galotto J, Guccio JG, Higgins GA, Ortega LG, West WH, Recant L. Necrolytic migratory erythema, presenting as candidiasis, due to a pancreatic glucagonoma. Cancer. 1979;44(2):558–63.

Kheir SM, Omura EF, Grizzle WE, Herrera GA, Lee I. Histologic variation in the skin lesions of the glucagonoma syndrome. Am J Surg Pathol. 1986;10(7):445–53.

Kiziltan ME, Benbir G, Akalin MA. Is diabetic dermopathy a sign for severe neuropathy in patients with diabetes mellitus? Nerve conduction studies and symptom analysis. Clin Neurophysiol. 2006;117(8):1862–9.

Kovacs RK, Korom I, Dobozy A, Farkas G, Ormos J, Kemeny L. Necrolytic migratory erythema. J Cutan Pathol. 2006;33(3):242–5.

Kreuter A, Knierim C, Stücker M, Pawlak F et al. Fumaric acid esters in necrobiosis lipoidica: results of a prospective, non-controlled study. Br J Dermatol. 2005;153 (4):802–7

Lamba S, Krishtul A, Tan MH, Lebwohl MG. Acanthosis nigricans in a plaque of scleredema on the back of a diabetic patient: a case report. Int J Dermatol. 2005;44(1):45–7.

Lee AY, Chey WY, Choi J, Jeon JS. Insulin-induced drug eruptions and reliability of skin tests. Acta Derm Venereol. 2002;82(2):114–7.

Linana JJ, Montoro FJ, Hernandez MD, Basomba A. Adverse reactions to insulin. An Med Interna. 1997;14(7):369–72.

Long CC, Laidler P, Holt PJ. Suprabasal acantholysis–an unusual feature of necrolytic migratory erythema. Clin Exp Dermatol. 1993;18(5):464–7.

Lopez X, Castells M, Ricker A, Velazquez EF, Mun E, Goldfine AB. Human insulin analog–induced lipoatrophy. Diabetes Care. 2008;31(3):442–4.

Mallinson CN, Bloom SR, Warin AP, Salmon PR, Cox B. A glucagonoma syndrome. Lancet. 1974;2(7871):1–5.

Marinkovich MP, Botella R, Datloff J, Sangueza OP. Necrolytic migratory erythema without glucagonoma in patients with liver disease. J Am Acad Dermatol. 1995;32(4):604–9.

McFadden N, Ree K, Søyland E, Larsen TE. Scleredema adultorum associated with a monoclonal gammopathy and generalized hyperpigmentation. Arch Dermatol. 1987;123(5):629–32.

McIntosh BC, Lahinjani S, Narayan D. Necrobiosis lipoidica resulting in squamous cell carcinoma. Conn Med. 2005;69(7):401–3.

Mendonca DA, Cosker T, Makwana NK. Vacuum-assisted closure to aid wound healing in foot and ankle surgery. Foot Ankle Int. 2005;26(9):761–6.

Mullans EA, Cohen PR. Iatrogenic necrolytic migratory erythema: a case report and review of nonglucagonoma-associated necrolytic migratory erythema. J Am Acad Dermatol. 1998;38 (5 Pt 2):866–73.

Ngo BT, Hayes KD, DiMiao DJ, Srinivasan SK, Huerter CJ, Rendell MS. Manifestations of cutaneous diabetic microangiopathy. Am J Clin Dermatol. 2005;6(4):225–37.

Nguyen K, Washenik K, Shupack J. Necrobiosis lipoidica diabeticorum treated with chloroquine. J Am Acad Dermatol. 2002;46(2 Suppl Case Reports):S34–6.

Ossowski B, Baum C. Das Pseudoglucagonom-Syndrome. Hautarzt. 1995;46(3):173–6.

Parmar RC, Bavdekar SB, Bansal S, Doraiswamy A, Khambadkone S. Scleredema adultorum. J Postgrad Med. 2000;46(2):91–3.

Perniciaro C, Rappaport KD, White JW Jr. Apoptosis with positive direct immunofluorescence findings in a patient with necrolytic migratory erythema. Cutis. 1998;62(3):129–32.

Pinzur M, Freeland R, Juknelis D. The association between body mass index and foot disorders in diabetic patients. Foot Ankle Int. 2005;26(5):375–7.

Radermecker RP, Piérard GE, Scheen AJ. Lipodystrophy reactions to insulin: effects of continuous insulin infusion and new insulin analogs. Am J Clin Dermatol. 2007;8(1):21–8.

Raile K, Noelle V, Landgraf R, Schwarz HP. Insulin antibodies are associated with lipoatrophy but also with lipohypertrophy in children and adolescents with type 1 diabetes. Exp Clin Endocrinol Diabet. 2001;109(8):393–6.

Rallis E, Korfitis C, Gregoriou S, Rigopoulos D. Assigning new roles to topical tacrolimus. Expert Opin Investig Drugs. 2007;16(8):1267–76.

Ramos AJ, Farias MA. Human insulin-induced lipoatrophy: a successful treatment with glucocorticoid. Diabetes Care. 2006;29(4):926–7.

Rappersberger K, Wolff-Schreiner E, Konrad K, Wolff K. Das Glucagonom-Syndrom. Hautarzt. 1987;38(10):589–98.

Richardson T, Kerr D. Skin-related complications of insulin therapy: epidemiology and emerging management strategies. Am J Clin Dermatol. 2003;4(10):661–7.

Robbins JM. Treatment of onychomycosis in the diabetic patient population. J Diabetes Complications. 2003;17(2):98–104.

Romano G, Moretti G, Di Benedetto A, Giofre C, Di Cesare E, Russo G, Califano L, Cucinotta D. Skin lesions in diabetes mellitus: prevalence and clinical correlations. Diabetes Res Clin Pract. 1998;39(2):101–6.

Shemer A, Bergman R, Linn S, Kantor Y, Friedman-Birnbaum R. Diabetic dermopathy and internal complications in diabetes mellitus. Int J Dermatol. 1998;37(2):113–5.

Shimizu I, Furuya K, Osawa H, Fujii Y, Makino H. 10a-65: a case of insulin-induced localized lobular panniculitis with evidence for the phagocytosis of insulin by histiocytes. Endocr J. 2007;54(3):477–80.

Smith AP, Doolas A, Staren ED. Rapid resolution of necrolytic migratory erythema after glucagonoma resection. J Surg Oncol. 1996;61(4):306–9.

Tanner M, Brasch J, Christophers E. Erythema necroticans migrans ohne Glucagonom. Hautarzt. 1994;45(7):480–3.

Technau K, Renkl A, Norgauer J, Ziemer M. Necrolytic migratory erythema with myelodysplastic syndrome without glucagonoma. Eur J Dermatol. 2005;15(2):110–2.

Tierney EP, Badger J. Etiology and pathogenesis of necrolytic migratory erythema: review of the literature. MedGenMed. 2004;6(3):4.

Tokura Y, Mizushima Y, Hata M, Takigawa M. Necrobiosis lipoidica of the glans penis. J Am Acad Dermatol. 2003;49(5):921–4.

Tom WL, Peng DH, Allaei A, Hsu D, Hata TR. The effect of short-contact topical tretinoin therapy for foot ulcers in patients with diabetes. Arch Dermatol. 2005;141(11):1373–7.

Truhan AP, Roenigk Jr. HH. The cutaneous mucinoses. J Am Acad Dermatol. 1986;14(1):1–18.

Tuchinda C, Kerr HA, Taylor CR, Jacobe H, Bergamo BM, Elmets C, Rivard J, Lim HW. UVA1 phototherapy for cutaneous diseases: an experience of 92 cases in the United States. Photodermatol Photoimmunol Photomed. 2006;22(5):247–53.

van Beek AP, de Haas ER, van Vloten WA, Lips CJ, Roijers JF, Canninga-van Dijk MR. The glucagonoma syndrome and necrolytic migratory erythema: a clinical review. Eur J Endocrinol. 2004;151(5):531–7.

Venencie PY, Powell FC, Su WP, Perry HO. Scleredema: a review of thirty-three cases. J Am Acad Dermatol. 1984;11(1):128–34.

Vijayasingam SM, Thai AC, Chan HL. Non-infective skin associations of diabetes mellitus. Ann Acad Med Singapore. 1988;17(4):526–35.

Wee SA, Possick P. Necrobiosis lipoidica. Dermatol Online J. 2004;10(3):18.

Wermers RA, Fatourechi V, Wynne AG, Kvols LK, Lloyd RV. The glucagonoma syndrome. Clinical and pathologic features in 21 patients. Medicine (Baltimore). 1996;75(2):53–63.

Wigington G, Ngo B, Rendell M. Skin blood flow in diabetic dermopathy. Arch Dermatol. 2004;140(10):1248–50.

Wonders J, Eekhoff EM, Heine R, Bruynzeel DP, Rustemeyer T. Insulin allergy: background, diagnosis and treatment. Ned Tijdschr Geneeskd. 2005;149(50):2783–8.

Yokoyama H, Fukumoto S, Koyama H, Emoto M, Kitagawa Y, Nishizawa Y. Insulin allergy; desensitization with crystalline zinc-insulin and steroid tapering. Diabetes Res Clin Pract. 2003;61(3):161–6.

Yosipovitch G, Hodak E, Vardi P, Shraga I, Karp M, Sprecher E, David M. The prevalence of cutaneous manifestations in IDDM patients and their association with diabetes risk factors and microvascular complications. Diabetes Care. 1998;21(4):506–9.

Obesity

11

Synopsis

> Obesity is defined as an increase of BMI above 30. It is frequently part of the metabolic syndrome (insulin-resistance syndrome). Adipocytokines play an important role in obesity-associated metabolic complications and support chronic inflammatory diseases. There is profound clinical data describing an association between obesity and psoriasis vulgaris. Other skin diseases observed in association with obesity are: Acanthosis nigricans (up to 74% of patients), acrochordons (skin tags), hirsutism (in females), keratosis pilaris, chronic venous insufficiency, lymphedema, piezogenic pedal papules, plantar hyperkeratosis (most common), striae distensae (stretch marks) as well as various infections such as intertrigo, candidosis, tinea pedis and cellulitis.

Aetiopathogenesis. Obesity is defined as an increase of BMI above 30. It is frequently part of the metabolic syndrome, which includes additionally increased levels of triglycerides, low level of HDL-C, increased blood pressure and increased fasting glucose (Table 11.1). Insulin resistance appears to underlie the features of the metabolic syndrome as a common pathogenesis; thus it is designated also as insulin-resistance syndrome (IRS) in the most recent literature. In IRS, target cells fail to respond to usual levels of circulating insulin. As a consequence, the insulin secretion is enhanced in order to maintain normoglycaemia. Compensatory hyperinsulinaemia due to enhanced β-cell secretion is an obligate accompanying feature in IRS. The overall prevalence of IRS reported is 10–25%. IRS originates from genetic factors and environmental factors such as increased food intake, reduced physical activity, aging and smoking. Moreover, several drugs are able to induce IRS, such as thiazide diuretics, β-adrenergic antagonists and glucocorticoids (Mlinar et al. 2007).

Intra-abdominal fat is not an inactive deposit, but it acts as an endocrine organ, which secretes several kinds of bioactive proteins (adipocytokines) promoting inflammation and

Walter K. H. Krause, *Cutaneous Manifestations of Endocrine Diseases*,
DOI: 10.1007/978-3-540-88367-8, © Springer-Verlag Berlin Heidelberg 2009

Table 11.1 Clinical identification of the metabolic syndrome as defined by the american heart association

Abdominal obesity (measured as waist circumference)	>102 cm in men, > 88 cm in women
Triglycerides	>150 mg dL^{-1}
HDL-C	<40 mg dL^{-1} in men, < 50 mg dL^{-1} in women
Blood pressure	>130/≥85 mm Hg
Fasting glucose	>100 mg dLb^{-1}

affecting glucose metabolism and vascular endothelial biology. Among the adipocytokines are IL-6, TNF-α, adiponectin and plasminogen activator inhibitor type 1 (PAI-1). Most recent studies indicate that adipocytokines play an important role in obesity-associated metabolic complications and suggest that chronically elevated local or systemic concentrations of adipocytokines contribute to the development of complications associated with obesity and IRS (Bulló et al. 2007; Sterry et al. 2007). From this point of view, insulin resistance is increasingly recognized as a chronic, low-level, inflammatory state with chronically increased levels of mainly TNF-α and IL-6 (Fernández-Real and Ricart 2003; Ritchie and Connell 2007).

Thus chronic inflammatory diseases are supported; e. g. rheumatoid arthritis and psoriasis. Incidence data on the association of psoriasis and obesity give evidence for a common pathogenesis of the two conditions. The chronic low-level inflammation may contribute to the extent of psoriatic lesions in obese patients (Hamminga et al. 2006; Sommer et al. 2006).

Obesity is a multigenic disease. Some monogenic forms of obesity were described, but the vast majority of obesity cases result from polygenic interactions. The products of two genes are known to have direct effects on the skin leptin and proopiomelanocortin (POMC); their contribution to the pathogenesis of common obesity, however, is unclear (Yosipovitch et al. 2007).

Cutaneous Manifestations. In 100 subsequent patients of a specialist nutrition clinic in Scotland, 75 claimed cutaneous problems. The most relevant problems were itchiness and dry skin, predominantly in groins, limbs and submammary folds (Brown et al. 2004).

Also various other dermatologic features may be associated with obesity (Table 11.2). The incidence of the disorders is closely associated with the severity of obesity.

Acanthosis nigricans is mentioned in a separate chapter (Chap. 12).

Acrochordons or skin tags (Fig. 11.1) are very common skin lesions; their etiopathogenesis is unclear. Their frequent occurrence also as a symptom in acromegaly (see Chap. 2) indicates a role of growth factors. This concerns keratosis pilaris too. Pathohistologically, the epidermis shows papillomatous hyperplasia occasionally with pseudo-horncysts (Fig. 11.2). The connective tissue is composed of loosely arranged collagen with a normal amount of elastic fibres (Adams and Mutasim 1999) and is well vascularized. As additional components, clusters of fat cells and a dermal melanocytic nevus have been observed.

Hirsutism is frequently associated with polycystic ovar syndrome (see Sect. 7.2).

Adiposis dolorosa (Dercum's disease) is characterized by multiple, painful, subcutaneous lipomas in obese, postmenopausal women. The painful lipomas are symmetrically distributed

Table 11.2 Skin disorders observed in obesity (compiled from Tyler et al. 2002; Scheinfeld 2004; Yosipovitch et al. 2007). See text for more details

Disorders associated with insulin resistance
Acanthosis nigricans (up to 74% of patients)
Acrochordons (skin tags)
Hirsutism and hyperandrogenism in females
Keratosis pilaris
Disorders due to mechanical factors
Adiposis dolorosa
Cellulité
Chronic venous insufficiency
Lymphedema
Piezogenic pedal papules
Plantar hyperkeratosis (most common)
Pressure ulcers
Striae distensae (stretch marks)
Disorders due to infections
Intertrigo
Candidosis
Tinea pedis (dermatomycosis)
Cellulitis
Necrotizing cellulitis/fasciitis (rare)
Gas gangrene (rare)
Inflammatory disorders
Atopic dermatitis
Androgenetic alopecia
Psoriasis

and are either diffuse or localized. Lower extremities, especially around the knees, are the most commonly involved sites. Pain increases on light pressure. The etiology is unknown; however, a metabolic or autoimmune mechanism was suspected to be involved (Yosipovitch et al. 2007).

Chronic venous insufficiency and lymphedema due to reduced flow within the veins and lymph vessels are more frequent in adipose individuals than in those with normal BMI.

Piezogenic papules (piezo means originating from pressure) are small, painful or asymptomatic papules of subcutaneous fat, which protrude (herniate) into the papillary stratum of the dermis. Piezogenic pedal papules were first described in 1968 as "herniation of fat" by Shelley and Rawnsley (1968). The papules appear to represent the peripheral fat chambers, which are part of the structure of the normal heel. The normal heel consists of a large cushion of fat, which is subdivided by trabecles of connective tissue (Grant and Gomez 1970; Woodrow et al. 1997; Schlapper et al. 1997). Piezogenic papules are very common, non-hereditary and usually are not the result of inherent connective tissue defect. They are rarely visible, but mainly palpable resembling bell buttons. The papules become apparent when an individual stands with full weight on the heels, and they resolve when the weight is removed. They occur predominantly over the medial and lateral aspects of the heels usually bilaterally (Fig. 11.3). Similar papules arise on the volar wrists when pressure

11

Fig. 11.1 Skin tags (acrochordons) in
adipositas. Soft, skin-coloured pending
tumours in the flexures, predominantly
in the axillae

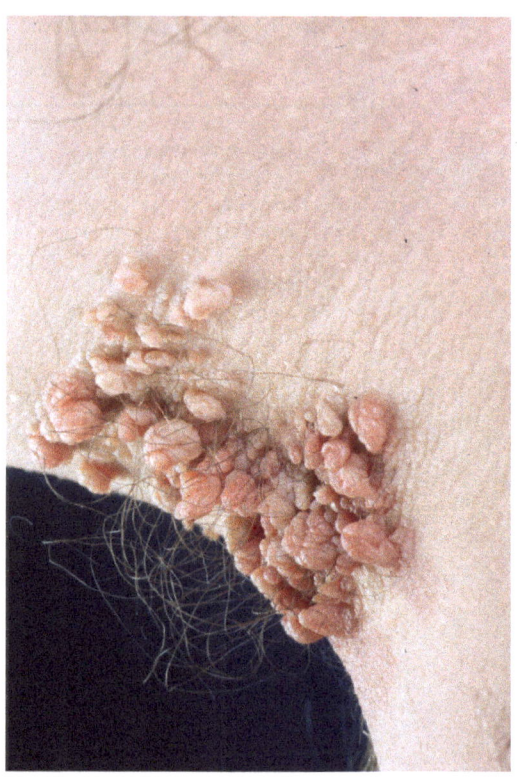

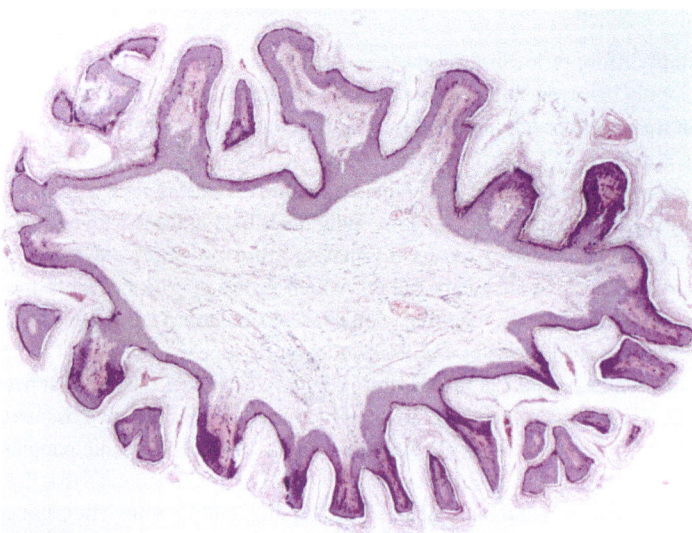

Fig. 11.2 Skin tags (acrochordons), pathohistology. The epidermis shows papillomatous hyperplasia. The connective tissue is composed of loosely arranged collagen and is well vascularized

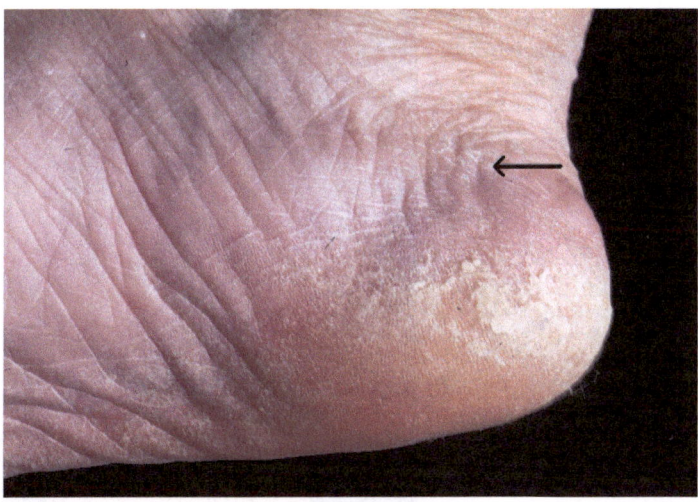

Fig. 11.3 Piezogenic papules in adipositas. They are often not visible, but palpable resembling bell buttons (arrow). The papules become apparent when an individual stands with full weight on the heels, and they resolve when the weight is removed

is applied; the first description of piezogenic wrist papules was presented by Laing and Fleischer (1991). In addition to obesity, vigorous physical activity may contribute to the development of piezogenic papules (Kohn and Blasi 1972).

Plantar hyperkeratosis was the most common dermatological manifestation in patients who weighed 76–100% more than their ideal body weight (Fig. 11.4). The use of insoles fitted by an orthotist helps lessen the symptoms (Hahler 2006).

Pressure ulcers: Several studies have demonstrated that obesity is associated with significant changes in cutaneous microcirculation and macrocirculation (Yosipovitch et al. 2007). Patients with obesity are at risk for pressure ulcers. Pressure ulcers typically develop over bony prominences; additionally, pressure in obese individuals is created when skin folds touch another, which may lead to pressure ulcers at unusual places (Hahler 2006). Pressure ulcers at a special site, the sole, are strongly correlated to the degree of obesity (Pinzur et al. 2005). However, elderly patients with obesity may have a reduced risk of pressure ulcers when compared to those with low weight (RR 0.7, 95% CI 0.4–1.0) (Compher et al. 2007).

Striae distensae are similar to those occurring in hypercortisolism (see Sects. 5.1 and 5.3).

Intertrigo is frequent in obesity (Fig. 11.5). The erosions result from the rubbing of the skin folds in conjunction. An augmentation of the physiologic bacterial and fungal flora plays a role. The erosions also favour superinfection with candida species inducing candidosis.

Tinea pedis (dermatomycosis) is also a typical infection associated with obesity.

Cellulitis and erysipelas are typical co-morbid conditions associated with obesity. Cinically, erythema, warmth, edema and fever are typical features (Fig. 11.6). Erysipelas occurs particularly in elderly individuals. The incidence in men and women does not differ significantly. A number of co-morbidities increases the risk of erysipelas, among them

Fig. 11.4 Plantar hyperkeratosis is the most common dermatological manifestation in obese patients

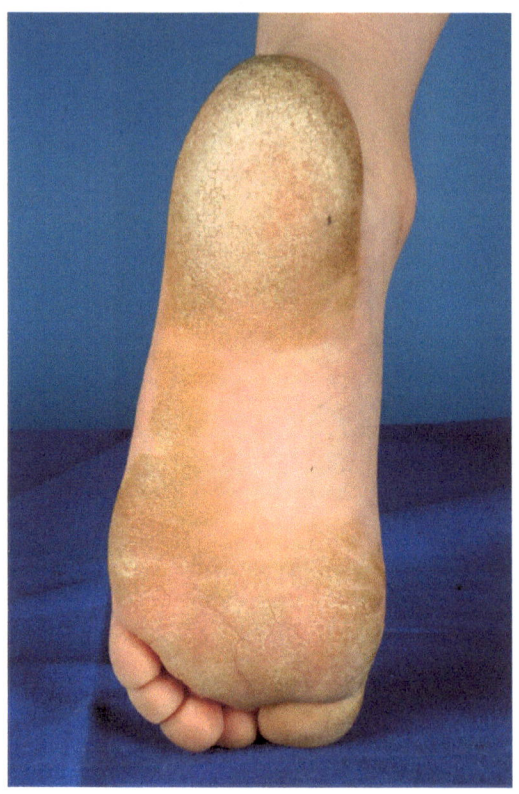

that with the highest risk is skin ulcer 7.34 (95% CI 1.77–30.52), while the next highest risk is obesity (4.10; 95% CI 2.01–8.36). The risk of recurrent erysipelas is enhanced also by strictly local diseases such as dermatomycosis and phlebitis (Bartholomeeusen et al. 2007). Cellulitis is usually caused by beta hemolytic streptococci; *S. aureus*, *Hemophilus influenza* and methicillin-resistant *S. aureus* (MRSA) were also observed.

Androgenetic alopecia was found also to be associated with obesity. Among 727 men (25–34 years of age), those with moderate to extensive androgenetic alopecia (17%) had a higher body mass index than those with little to no alopecia ($p < 0.05$) (Hirsso et al. 2007).

Atopic diseases were found to be a risk factor for obesity (Silva et al. 2007). Among 228 children, the authors observed 112 children with atopic diseases (75.9% asthma, 21.4% rhinitis and 2.7% eczema) and 116 children without atopy. The median age was 10.5 and 10.3 years, respectively. The prevalence of overweight or obesity was significantly greater in the atopic group (44.6% vs 31.9%, p 0.05). No sex differences could be calculated.

Psoriasis vulgaris: There is profound clinical data describing an association between obesity and the metabolic syndrome and psoriasis vulgaris, in particular with plaque psoriasis (Fig. 11.7; Puig-Sanz 2007). Naldi et al. (1999) demonstrated a higher prevalence of obesity in psoriasis patients than in non-psoriatic controls in the Italian case-control study (Table 11.3). Also in a study of the Utah department of dermatology, the psoriasis patients

Fig. 11.5 Intertrigo in adipositas. Erosions in the large skin folds (groins, axillae, submammary) resulting from the rubbing of the skin areas in conjunction

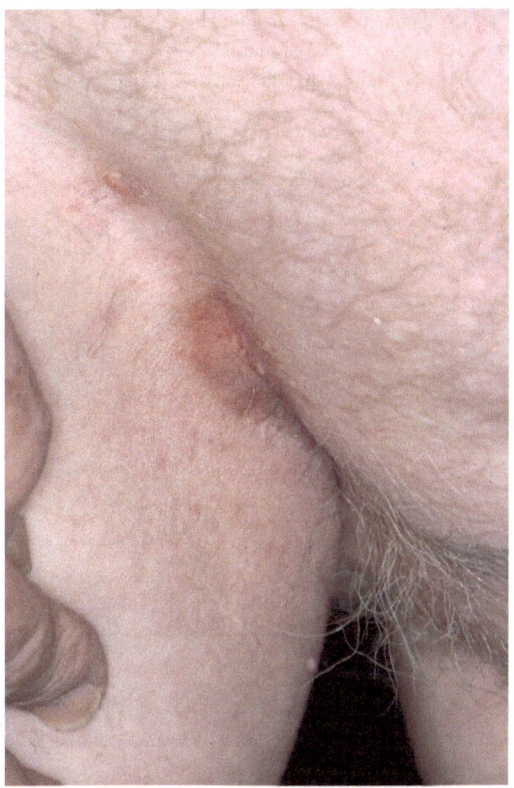

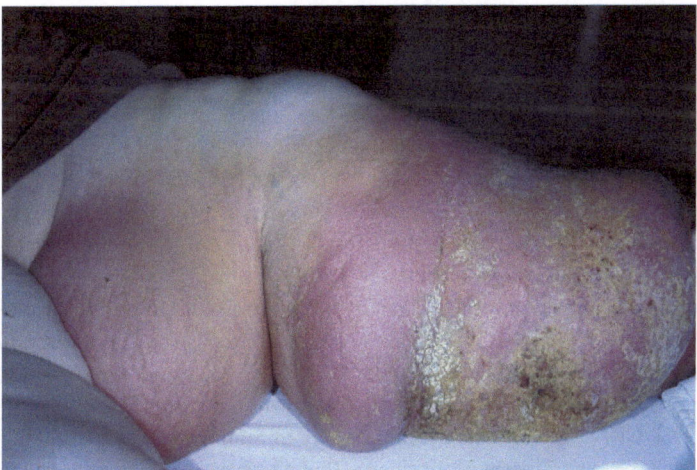

Fig. 11.6 Cellulitis in severe adipositas. The patient demonstrated here had many relapses of the disease, she developed a severe lymphedema. All trials to reduce weight failed

Fig. 11.7 Plaque psoriasis in adipositas. A circumscribed, red plaque
is covered with loosely adherent,
silvery scales

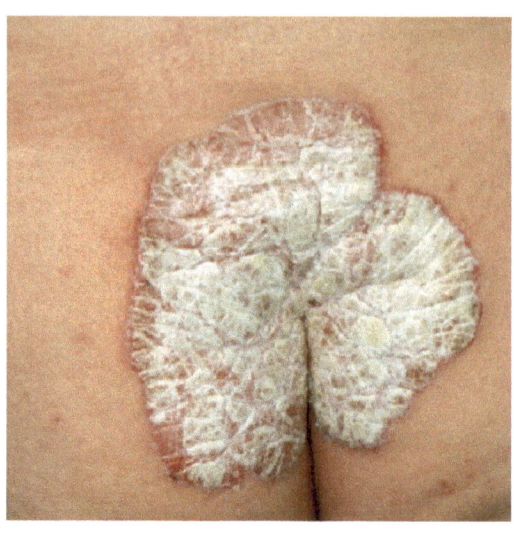

Table 11.3 Body mass index in patients with psoriasis and non-psoriatic individuals (Naldi
et al. 1999)

Body mass index, kg/m^2	Psoriasis patients	Control patients	Significance
<22.0	103 (25.6%)	214 (34.7%)	
22.0–26.0	159 (39.4%)	247 (40.1%)	
>26.0	141 (35.0%)	155 (25.2%)	12.7 (.001)

had a higher prevalence of obesity than non-psoriatic control patients. Psoriasis inversa
was more frequent in obese patients (5% of non-obese, 11% of obese and 13% of morbidly
obese patients). The authors point out that the profound adverse effect of psoriasis on an
individual's physical, social and mental well-being may play a role in the origin of obesity (Herron et al. 2005). In a cross-sectional study of 127,706 patients with mild psoriasis
and 3,854 with severe psoriasis, diabetes, hypertension, hyperlipidemia and obesity had a
higher prevalence in severe psoriasis than in mild psoriasis and controls. The odds ratio to
be obese was 1.79 (95% CI 1.55–2.05) in severe psoriasis as compared to controls (Neimann et al. 2006). Gisondi et al. (2007) found the metabolic syndrome significantly more
frequent in psoriatic patients older than 40 years than in controls (30.1% vs. 20.6%, OR
1.65, 95% CI 1.16–2.35; $P = 0.005$). In the study of Sommer et al. (2006), the increased
OR for metabolic syndrome in psoriasis was found to start at mid age (40–49 years) and
to persist throughout further life. The effect was aggravated by other risk factors related to
lifestyle, e.g. smoking and alcohol consumption, which are also associated with psoriasis.
As an illustrative example of the association, de Menezes Ettinger et al. (2006) described a
severely obese 56-year-old man (BMI 46.9) suffering from psoriasis, who had lost 34.8%

Table 11.4 Therapeutic regimen for specific complications of obesity (from Garcia Hidalgo 2002; Hahler 2006)

Disease	Treatment
Acanthosis nigricans due to insulin resistance	Vitamin D3 analogues
Skin tags	Surgical
Hirsutism	Antiandrogens, contraceptives
Striae	No treatment known, laser were applied for blanching
Lymphedema	Weight reduction
Cellulitis	Antibiotics specific for bacteria
Chronic venous insufficiency	Phlebologic surgery
Pressure ulcers	Treatment schedules of chronic wounds
Intertrigo and candidosis	Antimycotics

of excess weight after performing an open gastric and presented with complete remission of the psoriasis without medication at 4 months follow-up.

Treatment: First and foremost, the treatment of skin disorders in obesity requires the treatment of obesity by restricted calorie intake, weight reduction and physical activity (Mlinar et al. 2007). In addition, there are specific therapeutic regimens for the complications described (Table 11.4).

The existing association of psoriasis and obesity and metabolic syndrome or IRS has also to be taken in account when choosing a psoriasis treatment. Therapeutic interventions for psoriasis by use of anti-inflammatory drugs including methotrexate (MTX) and TNFα antagonists appear to lower the risk of aggravation of IRS (Hamminga et al. 2006; Mrowietz et al. 2006; Sommer et al. 2006; Kremers et al. 2007; Sterry et al. 2007; Wakkee et al. 2007).

References

Adams BB, Mutasim DF. Elastic tissue in fibroepithelial polyps. Am J Dermatopathol. 1999; 21(5):446–8.
Bartholomeeusen S, Vandenbroucke J, Truyers C, Buntinx F. Epidemiology and comorbidity of erysipelas in primary care. Dermatology. 2007;215(2):118–22.
Brown J, Wimpenny P, Maughan H. Skin problems in people with obesity. Nurs Stand. 2004; 18(35):38–42.
Bulló M, Casas-Agustench P, Amigó-Correig P, Aranceta J, Salas-Salvadó J. Inflammation, obesity and comorbidities: the role of diet. Public Health Nutr. 2007;10(10A):1164–72.
Compher C, Kinosian BP, Ratcliffe SJ, Baumgarten M. Obesity reduces the risk of pressure ulcers in elderly hospitalized patients. J Gerontol A Biol Sci Med Sci. 2007;62(11):1310–2.
de Menezes Ettinger JE, Azaro E, de Souza CA, dos Santos Filho PV, Mello CA, Neves M Jr, de Amaral PC, Fahel E. Remission of psoriasis after open gastric bypass. Obes Surg. 2006;16(1):94–7. emedicine (Update 11-29-2007 by Stephen W White)

Fernández-Real JM, Ricart W. Insulin resistance and chronic cardiovascular inflammatory syndrome. Endocr Rev. 2003;24(3):278–301.

Garcia Hidalgo L. Dermatological complications of obesity. Am J Clin Dermatol. 2002;3(7):497–506.

Gisondi P, Tessari G, Conti A, Piaserico S, Schianchi S, Peserico A, Giannetti A, Girolomoni G. Prevalence of metabolic syndrome in patients with psoriasis: a hospital-based case-control study. Br J Dermatol. 2007;157(1):68–73.

Grant DJ, Gomez F. Piezogenic pedal papules. Arch Dermatol. 1970;101(5):619–20.

Hahler B. An overview of dermatological conditions commonly associated with the obese patient. Ostomy Wound Manage. 2006;52(6):34–6, 38, 40.

Hamminga EA, van der Lely AJ, Neumann HA, Thio HB. Chronic inflammation in psoriasis and obesity: implications for therapy. Med Hypotheses. 2006;67(4):768–73.

Herron MD, Hinckley M, Hoffman MS, Papenfuss J, Hansen CB, Callis KP, Krueger GG. Impact of obesity and smoking on psoriasis presentation and management. Arch Dermatol. 2005;141(12):1527–34.

Hirsso P, Rajala U, Hiltunen L, Jokelainen J, Keinänen-Kiukaanniemi S, Näyhä S. Obesity and low-grade inflammation among young Finnish men with early-onset alopecia. Dermatology. 2007;214(2):125–9.

Kohn SR, Blasi JM. Piezogenic pedal papules. Arch Dermatol. 1972;106(4):597–8.

Kremers HM, McEvoy MT, Dann FJ, Gabriel SE. Heart disease in psoriasis. J Am Acad Dermatol. 2007;57(2):347–54.

Laing VB, Fleischer AB Jr. Piezogenic wrist papules: a common and asymptomatic finding. J Am Acad Dermatol. 1991;24(3):415–7.

Mlinar B, Marc J, Janez A, Pfeifer M. Molecular mechanisms of insulin resistance and associated diseases. Clin Chim Acta. 2007;375(1–2):20–35.

Mrowietz U, Elder JT, Barker J. The importance of disease associations and concomitant therapy for the long-term management of psoriasis patients. Arch Dermatol Res. 2006;298(7):309–19.

Naldi L, Peli L, Parazzini F, et al. Association of early-stage psoriasis with smoking and male alcohol consumption: Evidence from an Italian case–control study. Arch Dermatol. 1999;135:1479–84

Neimann AL, Shin DB, Wang X, Margolis DJ, Troxel AB, Gelfand JM. Prevalence of cardiovascular risk factors in patients with psoriasis. J Am Acad Dermatol. 2006;55(5):829–35.

Pinzur M, Freeland R, Juknelis D. The association between body mass index and foot disorders in diabetic patients. Foot Ankle Int. 2005;26(5):375–7.

Puig-Sanz L. Psoriasis, a systemic disease? Actas Dermosifiliogr. 2007;98(6):396–402.

Ritchie SA, Connell JM. The link between abdominal obesity, metabolic syndrome and cardiovascular disease. Nutr Metab Cardiovasc Dis. 2007;17(4):319–26.

Scheinfeld NS. Obesity and dermatology. Clin Dermatol. 2004;22(4):303–9.

Shelley WB, Rawnsley HM. Painful feet due to herniation of fat. JAMA. 1968;205:308–9

Silva MJ, Ribeiro MC, Carvalho F, Gonçalves Oliveira JM. Atopic disease and body mass index. Allergol Immunopathol. 2007;35(4):130–5.

Sommer DM, Jenisch S, Suchan M, Christophers E, Weichenthal M. Increased prevalence of the metabolic syndrome in patients with moderate to severe psoriasis. Arch Dermatol Res. 2006;298(7):321–8.

Sterry W, Strober BE, Menter A. on behalf of the International Psoriasis Council. Obesity in psoriasis: the metabolic, clinical and therapeutic implications. Report of an interdisciplinary conference and review. Br J Dermatol. 2007;157(4):649–55.

Tyler I, Wiseman MC, Crawford RI, Birmingham CL. Cutaneous manifestations of eating disorders. J Cutan Med Surg. 2002;6(4):345–53.

Wakkee M, Thio HB, Prens EP, Sijbrands EJ, Neumann HA. Unfavorable cardiovascular risk profiles in untreated and treated psoriasis patients. Atherosclerosis. 2007;190(1):1–9.

Woodrow SL, Brereton-Smith G, Handfield-Jones S. Painful piezogenic pedal papules: response
to local electro-acupuncture. Br J Dermatol. 1997;136(4):628–30.

Yosipovitch G, DeVore A, MD, Dawn A. Obesity and the skin: Skin physiology and skin manifestations of obesity. J Am Acad Dermatol. 2007;56:901–16.

Intestinal Hormones

Synopsis

Acanthosis Nigricans

> Acanthosis nigricans (AN) is due to the hyperactivity of different growth factors such as EGF, FGF and IGF, inducing hyperplasia of keratinocytes. AN is a feature of insulin resistance, of obesity and of malignant tumours, mainly in the gastrointestinal tract. The lesions of AN are grey–brown to black, rough with prominent skin lines and occur most commonly in flexural areas. The clinical feature is uniform in all causes, thus the classification of AN as malignant and benign types is not justified. The treatment of the underlying disease is essential. For treatment skin abradation, calcipotriol and laser therapy have been recommended.

Carcinoid Syndrome

> Carcinoid syndrome is caused by an excessive secretion of serotonin from carcinoid tumours, mostly localized in the small intestine. Serotonin induces the typical flush, occurring in 85% of patients. It begins suddenly and lasts 20–30 s, primarily involving the face, neck and upper chest. Some patients develop pellagra-like lesions due to the lack of tryptophan or sclerodermic lesions without Raynaud's phenomenon. The diagnosis of carcinoid syndrome is confirmed by the proof of increased urinary excretion of 5-hydroxyindol acetic acid. The treatment requires removal of the tumour. Flushing itself is completely abolished by somatostatin, but the treatment with glucocorticoids and beta-inhibitors is ineffective.

12.1
Acanthosis Nigricans

Aetiopathogenesis. Acanthosis (acantho meaning thorn) nigricans (black) is a rare disease due to the hyperactivity of different growth factors, inducing hyperplasia of keratinocytes. The hyperpigmentation observed appears to be secondary to acanthosis and papillomatosis

Walter K. H. Krause, *Cutaneous Manifestations of Endocrine Diseases*,
DOI: 10.1007/978-3-540-88367-8, © Springer-Verlag Berlin Heidelberg 2009

of the epidermis due to increased POMC production by keratinocytes, but direct evidence is lacking.

Acanthosis nigricans (AN) occurs in mutations of the receptors of epidermal growth factors (EGF) and the fibroblast growth factors (FGF) or by mutations of ligands themselves. In inherited syndromes with AN, inappropriate activation of the insulin-like growth factor (IGF)-1 receptor (IGF1R) and activating mutations of the epidermal growth factor (EGF) fibroblast growth factor (FGF) and their receptors have been shown. The growth factors are members of the tyrosine kinase (TK) receptor (TKR) superfamily. On a molecular basis, the common pathogenic pathway of the disease is the activation of tyrosin kinases, which exert mitogenic and antiapoptotic effects onto the keratinocytes (Torley et al. 2002).

An important cause of AN is insulin resistance. There is a statistically significant correlation of increasing severity of AN with increasing BMI and body fat percentage in patients with insulin resistance and diabetes, and is also known to occur in adolescents (Selkin et al. 2005; Bolding et al. 2005).

AN is often a symptom of a malignant tumour, mainly in the gastrointestinal tract, but other tumours have also been described, including adrenal, bile duct, bladder, breast, cervical, endometrium, hepatic, laryngeal, lung, lymphoid, ovarian, pituitary, prostate, renal, testicular, and thyroid, in addition to sarcomas (Mekhail and Markman 2002; Stone and Buescher 2005). AN may precede the clinical diagnosis of the tumour; it regresses after extirpation. It is unknown, however, whether a relapse of AN also indicates a relapse of the tumour. It has also been observed following bone marrow transplantation in lymphoblastic lymphoma; in this case it is likely to be the consequence of a graft-versus-host reaction.

Cutaneous Manifestations. The lesions of AN are grey–brown to black, rough, have thickened plaques and prominent skin lines, and occur most commonly in flexural areas (e.g. axillae, back and sides of neck, inguinal creases, infra-mammary) (Fig. 12.1). The intensity of skin changes depends on the skin colour (Lopez-Alvarenga et al. 2006). Also palms and soles show hyperplasia of the relief as 'tripe palms' (Fig. 12.2). AN is frequently asymptomatic, but patients may present with lesions that are painful, disfiguring, malodorous or macerated.

The clinical feature is uniform in all causes, thus the earlier used classification of AN as malignant and benign types is not justified.

Histopathologicy. There is papillomatosis with a thinned epidermis on the top of the finger-like papillae and mild acanthosis in the clefts with overlying hyperkeratosis. A non-specific inflammatory infiltrate in the superficial dermis is occasionally found, but is usually absent. The presence of keratin cysts may resemble a seborrhoic keratosis. As a differential diagnosis, epidermal nevi with the feature of AN have been reported, which were stable since childhood (Ersoy-Evans et al. 2006).

Treatment. Treatment of AN is difficult. The treatment of the underlying disease (obesity, diabetes mellitus, intestinal tumour) is essential. An improved control of hyperinsulinemia may help to control AN in these cases. Systemic treatments that have been reported to help clear AN include metformin, octreotide and retinoids (Hermanns-Le et al. 2004; Yosipovitch et al. 2007). Topically, skin abradation, calcipotriol and laser therapy have been recommended (Garcia Hidalgo 2002).

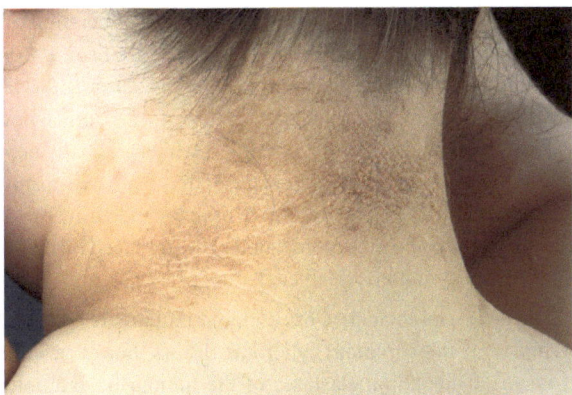

Fig. 12.1 Acanthosis nigricans. Gray-brown to black thickened plaques and prominent skin lines in the neck

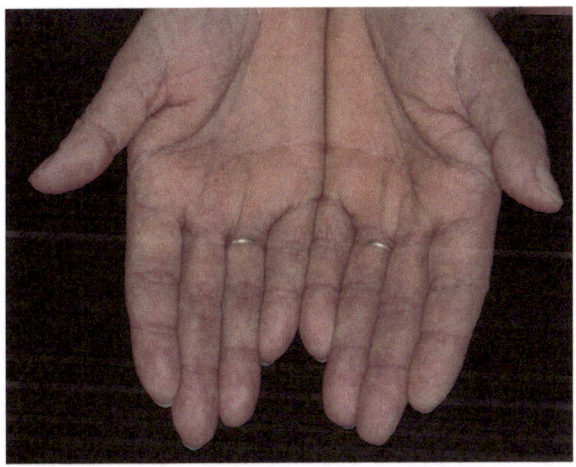

Fig. 12.2 Acanthosis nigricans. The palms show gray-brown hyperplasia of the relief as 'tripe palms'

12.2
Carcinoid Syndrome

Aetiopathogenesis. Carcinoid cells originate from the Kulchitsky cells of Lieberkuehns crypts (Glandulae intestinalis) of the small intestine. Although most carcinoid tumours originate from the small intestine, they can spread to large parts of the intestinum, the stomach and the bronchus; they may metastasize to lymph nodes and the liver (Sitaraman and Goldfinger 2005). However, primary tumours may also occur in the oesophagus, pancreas, liver, biliary tract, gallbladder and Meckel's diverticulum, in the ovary, in otolaryngeal organs and the breast (Modlin et al. 2005).

The pathophysiogical basis of the syndrome is an excessive secretion of serotonin and a malfunction of the tryptophan metabolism. In the normal metabolism, 1% of the daily intake of tryptophan is metabolized to serotonin, but in carcinoid syndrome this amount increases up to 60%. As a consequence, a tryptophan deficiency of other organs occurs. Serotonin induces vasoconstriction and dilation of the arterioles, which clinically appears as the typical flush. In addition, histamine, kallikrein, prostaglandins, some vasoactive peptides such as substance P and neurokinin A, and a wide range of neuroendocrine mediators dependent on the origin of the tumour have been demonstrated to be produced by the carcinoid tumour, which intensify the clinical symptoms (Bell et al. 2005; Jabbour et al. 2006).

Cutaneous Manifestations. The incidence of carcinoid tumours is approx. 1.5 per 100,000 of the population per year; the carcinoid syndrome occurs, however, in less than 10% of these patients. It occurs if hepatic metastases of the tumour or extraintestinal carcinoid tumours are present (Bell et al. 2005).

There are four main categories of cutaneous manifestations:

1. Episodic flushing is the clinical hallmark of the carcinoid syndrome and it occurs in 85% of patients (Bell et al. 2005; Fig. 12.3). The typical flush begins suddenly and lasts 20–30 s. It primarily involves the face, neck and upper chest. As subjective symptoms, the patients report mild burning sensation. Most flushing episodes occur spontaneously, but they can be provoked by eating, drinking alcohol, defecation, emotional events, palpation of the liver and by anaesthesia. With progress of the disease the episodes may last longer and the flushing may be more diffuse and cyanotic. The colour of the flushing may be pink to red in tumours originating in the stomach, lung and pancreas, or cyanotic in tumours originating from the midgut. The gastric carcinoid variant induces patchy, sharply demarcated, serpiginous and cherry red flushed with intense pruritus. In patients with the bronchial carcinoid variant, the flushes can be very severe and prolonged; they may last for hours or even days. The intestinal tumour produces the classical flushing as described above. Flushing in carcinoid syndrome is similar to the physiologic flushing, probably because of the common trigger mechanisms. Due to prolonged and repeated vasodilation, venous teleangiectasias may occur (Fig. 12.4). In the series of 25 patients described by Bell et al. (2005), three patients developed classical features of rosacea with facial erythema, telangiectasia and pustules, and two of them also had early rhinophyma. After years of flushing, features of rosacea may develop. The occurrence of rosacea indicates that possibly circulating vasodilators are involved in the pathogenesis of the disease. Also angioedema may be a consequence of carcinoid tumours. Rodriguez Trabado et al. (2004) reported Quincke oedema as a single manifestation of a bronchial carcinoid tumour.
2. Some patients develop pellagra-like lesions with pigmentation and hyperkeratosis in the legs or the arms (5/25 in the series of Bell et al. 2005; Fig. 12.5). The feature is related to a corresponding niacin deficiency in the syndrome, since up to 60% of dietary tryptophan is consumed (Sitaraman and Goldfinger 2005).

3. Sclerodermic lesions without Raynaud's phenomenon and the predominant involvement of the lower limb lesions are rare (2/25 patients of the series of Bell et al. 2005). Scleroderma has been exclusively associated with carcinoids of the gut. Histopathologically, in these cases the skin showed epidermal flattening of the rete ridges, lymphocytic infiltration of the dermis and enhancement of collagen depositions (Ratnavel et al. 1994; Pavlovic et al. 1995). The enhanced secretion of substance P or neurokinin from the tumour may stimulate of collagen synthesis, which are secreted only by this gut tumours, while serotonin appears to be of minor importance (Handley et al. 1993). Scleroderma has been related to poor prognosis of the disease, since it is often associated with fibrotic heart disease (Bell et al. 2005; Jabbour et al. 2006).
4. Metastasis of malignant carcinoid syndrome to the skin is a rare event. In a case reported by Archer et al. (1985), intestinal symptoms preceded the appearance of a nodule at the chin by 1 year. Only at the time of the detection of the skin lesion, was the diagnosis of carcinoid syndrome confirmed by increased 24-h urinary level of vanillylmandelic acid. Histopathologically, the nodule showed cellular aggregation in a thecal or trabecular arrangement and large numbers of fine argyrophil secretory granules.

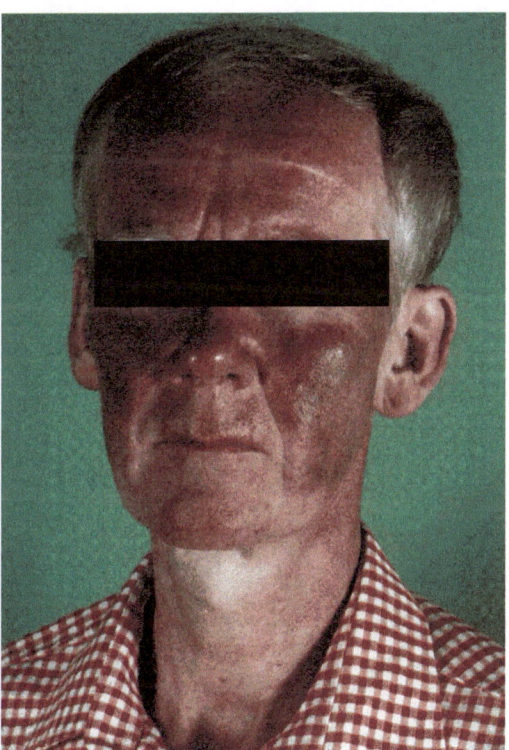

Fig. 12.3 Carcinoid syndrome. The typical flush, the clinical hallmark of the carcinoid syndrome, begins suddenly and lasts 20 to 30 seconds. It primarily involves the face, neck and upper chest. (Courtesy of Prof. Dr. Arnold, Marburg)

12

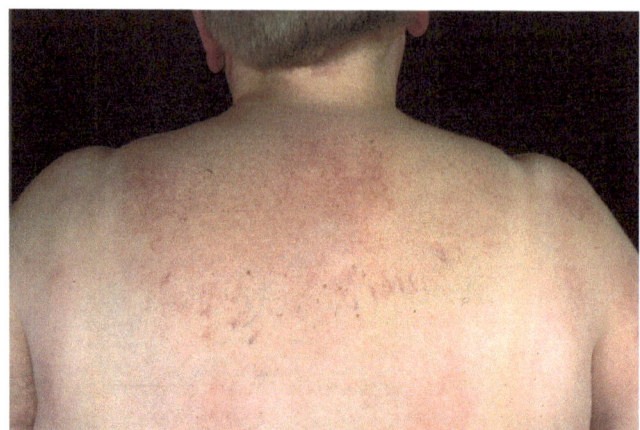

Fig. 12.4 Teleangiektasia in carcinoid syndrome. The skin shows telangiectasias in light-exposed areas of the upper back, which represent phlebectasias to the prolonged and repeated vasodilation due to the flushes

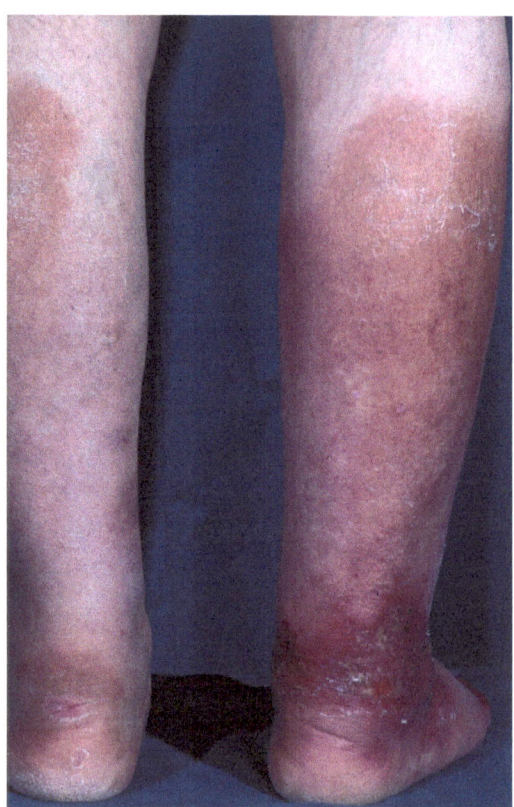

Fig. 12.5 Pellagroid in carcinoid syndrome. Diffuse, not sun-dependent pigmentation and hyperkeratosis

The diagnosis of carcinoid syndrome is confirmed by the proof of a maximally increased urinary excretion of 5-hydroxyindol acetic acid (5-HIAA) up to 1,000 mg per day (Sitaraman and Goldfinger 2005).

Histopathology. Sclerodermic skin changes in carcinoid syndrome show flattening of the epidermal rete ridges. There is an extensive deposition of collagen in the dermis, accompanied by a perivascular and periappendageal lymphocytic infiltrate (Green 1989; Ratnavel et al. 1994).

Treatment. The therapy of the syndrome requires removal of the tumour. If this is not possible, long-acting somatostatin analoges such as octreotide is the treatment of choice. Flushing is completely abolished by somatostatin. There are no cutaneous side effects of the treatment (Camisa 1989). Although a regression of skin symptoms has been reported, there was no remission of the tumour (Pavlovic et al. 1995). The treatment with glucocorticoids and beta-inhibitors does not improve the symptoms. A resolution of pruritus has been observed after treatment with glucocorticoids by Ratnavel et al. (1994), but the scleroderma remained unchanged.

References

Archer CB, Wells RS, MacDonald DM. Metastatic cutaneous carcinoid. J Am Acad Dermatol. 1985;13(2 Pt 2):363–6.

Bell HK, Poston GJ, Vora J, Wilson NJ. Cutaneous manifestations of the malignant carcinoid syndrome. Br J Dermatol. 2005;152(1):71–5.

Bolding J, Wratchford T, Perkins K, Ogershok P. Prevalence of obesity, acanthosis nigricans and hyperinsulinemia in an adolescent clinic. W V Med J. 2005;101(3):112–5.

Camisa C. Somatostatin and a long-acting analogue, octreotide acetate. Relevance to dermatology. Arch Dermatol. 1989;125(3):407–12.

Ersoy-Evans S, Sahin S, Mancini AJ, Paller AS, Guitart J. The acanthosis nigricans form of epidermal nevus. J Am Acad Dermatol. 2006;55(4):696–8.

Garcia Hidalgo L. Dermatological complications of obesity. Am J Clin Dermatol. 2002;3(7):497–506.

Green TPR. Scleroderma in association with carcinoid syndrome. Br J Dermatol. 1989;121(Suppl. 34):80.

Handley J, Walsh M, Armstrong K, Russell C, Buchanan K, Bingham A. Malignant carcinoid syndrome associated with cutaneous scleroderma. Br J Dermatol. 1993;129(2):222–3.

Jabbour SA, Davidovici BB, Wolf R. Rare syndromes. Clin Dermatol. 2006;24:299–316

Modlin IM, Shapiro MD, Kidd M. An analysis of rare carcinoid tumors: clarifying these clinical conundrums. World J Surg. 2005;29(1):92–101.

Pavlovic M, Saiag P, Lotz JP, Marinho E, Clerici T, Izrael V. Regression of sclerodermatous skin lesions in a patient with carcinoid syndrome treated by octreotide. Arch Dermatol. 1995;131(10):1207–9.

Ratnavel RC, Burrows NP, Pye RJ. Scleroderma and the carcinoid syndrome. Clin Exp Dermatol. 1994;19(1):83–5.

Rodriguez Trabado A, Riesco Miranda JA, Porcel Carreno S, Rodriguez Martin E, Fletes Peral C, Jimenez Timon S, Alvarado Arenas M, Hernandez Arbeiza J, Cobo Lopez R. Angioedema as a single manifestation of carcinoid syndrome in a bronchial carcinoid tumor. Allergol Immunopathol (Madr). 2004;32(4):235–7.

Sitaraman SV, Goldfinger ST: The carcinoid syndrome. Uptodate (13.2) June 2005. (www.utdol.com).

Hermanns-Le T, Scheen A, Pierard GE. Acanthosis nigricans associated with insulin resistance: pathophysiology and management. Am J Clin Dermatol. 2004;5(3):199–203.

Lopez-Alvarenga JC, García-Hidalgo L, Landa-Anell MV, Santos-Gómez R, González-Barranco J, Comuzzie A. Influence of skin color on the diagnostic utility of clinical acanthosis nigricans to predict insulin resistance in obese patients. Arch Med Res. 2006;37(6):744–8.

Mekhail TM, Markman M. Acanthosis nigricans with endometrial carcinoma: case report and review of the literature. Gynecol Oncol. 2002;84(2):332–4.

Selkin BA, Reynolds RV, Selkin G. Cutaneous manifestations of internal malignancy. UptoDate® 2005 (www.utdol.com).

Stone SP, Buescher LS. Life-threatening paraneoplastic cutaneous syndromes. Clin Dermatol. 2005;23:301–6.

Torley D, Bellus GA, Munro CS. Genes, growth factors and acanthosis nigricans. Br J Dermatol. 2002;147(6):1096–101.

Yosipovitch G, DeVore A, Dawn A. Obesity and the skin: skin physiology and skin manifestations of obesity. J Am Acad Dermatol. 2007;56(6):901–16; quiz 917–20.

Polyendocrine Disorders

13

Synopsis

Multiple Endocrine Neoplasias and Lichen Amyloidosus

> Patients with multiple endocrine neoplasia type 2A develop various endocrine
> tumours, most frequently thyroid carcinoma, pheochromocytoma and primary
> hyperparathyroidism. The typical skin disease is lichen amyloidosus, which is
> a pruritic dermatosis occurring largely in the pretibial and intrascapular areas.
> The amyloid found in the lesions originates from keratinocytes. Reports on the
> treatment of lichen amyloidosus with antihistamines, intralesional injection of
> glucocorticoids, etretinate, UVB irradiation and dermabrasion are published in
> the literature.

Autoimmune Polyendocrinopathy Syndrome Type I

> The autoimmune polyendocrinopathy syndrome type I (APS 1) is caused by
> mutations in the autoimmune regulator gene (AIRE), which influences induction
> of self-tolerance. APS 1 is characterized by the presence of two of three major
> clinical symptoms: Addison's disease, hypoparathyroidism and chronic muco-
> cutaneous candidiasis, which is usually the first manifestation of APS 1 seen
> even in childhood. Other infectious and autoimmune-induced skin lesions such
> as vitiligo and alopecia areata have also been described in case reports. Treat-
> ment regimen in the syndrome refers to the singular symptoms, e.g. systemic
> antimycotic treatment of candidosis.

13.1
Multiple Endocrine Neoplasias and Lichen Amyloidosus

Aetiopathogenesis. Lichen amyloidosus (LA) is a pruritic dermatosis occurring mainly
in the pretibial and intrascapular areas. The amyloid found in the lesions originates from
keratinocytes, which undergo filamentous degeneration (Masu et al. 1981; Breathnach

Walter K. H. Krause, *Cutaneous Manifestations of Endocrine Diseases*,
DOI: 10.1007/978-3-540-88367-8, © Springer-Verlag Berlin Heidelberg 2009

1988). Due to the similarity of the disease to lichen simplex chronicus, which is most likely induced by chronic scratching, and because in most patients the pruritus precedes the skin lesions, Weyers et al. (1997) as well as Salim et al. (2005) suggested that LA is a variant of lichen simplex chronicus in which scratching leads to the necrosis of keratinocytes and secondarily to the formation of amyloid in the papillary dermis.

LA is a typical skin disease of multiple endocrine neoplasia (MEN) 2A. MEN 2A is an inherited autosomal dominant disorder with very high penetrance. The genetic defect involves the RET proto-oncogene on chromosome 10, a receptor tyrosine kinase that transduces growth and differentiation signals in several tissues. Screening with molecular methods for the RET proto-oncogene permits an early diagnosis of the MEN-2 syndromes (OMIM). The patients develop different endocrine tumours, most frequently thyroid carcinoma, pheochromocytoma and primary hyperparathyroidism, but the conditions are not present in all the patients and can manifest at a distance of years (Verga et al. 2003). In different families with MEN 2A, the presence of LA was observed only in family members with manifest endocrine abnormalities, but it appeared to be independent of the kind of the tumour arising (Nunziata et al. 1989; Donovan et al. 1989; Robinson et al.1992; Bugalho et al. 1992; Modigliani et al. 1998; Gullu et al. 2005). For this reason, already Robinson et al. (1992) discussed whether the patients with and without LA represent different types of MEN 2A. Verga et al. (2003) reported that LA was present only in patients with the RET mutation involving cysteine in position 634. The RET ligand is related to a glial cell-line derived neurotropic factor, which may allow a hypothesis for the pathogenesis of LA in MEN 2A.

Chabre et al. (1992); Rivollier et al. (1999) and Verga et al. (2003) used the term notalgia paresthetica to describe the lesions of LA in MEN 2A. Notalgia paresthetica was believed to represent a peripheral nervous system disorder of the posterior dorsal nerves characterized by pruritus, paraesthesia and hyperaesthesia. It has been remarkable that pruritus and skin lesions were always located in the dermatomes between C4 and T5. Neurological examination usually failed to find any correlation between neural abnormalities and the presence of LA. The authors suggested that the cutaneous lesions were secondary to neural pathology and the amyloid as deposits of apoptotic keratinocytes was secondary to scratching. Possibly, notalgia paraestetica is based on a vertebral anomaly, but this assumption did not provide a satisfying explanation on its association with MEN 2A.

Cutaneous Manifestations. LA in MEN 2A is characterized by pruritic, scaly, papular and pigmented lesions, located in the interscapular region or on the extensor surfaces of the extremities. (Fig. 13.1). The first symptom is intense pruritus of the area. It improves with sun exposure and worsens during periods of stress. With persistence, the area develops hyperpigmented brown-coloured papules (Verga et al. 2003; Jabbour et al. 2006). In the five families examined by Robinson et al. (1992) 46% had unilateral and 64% bilateral pruritic and lichenoid skin lesions located over the upper back. MEN 2A was present in 97% of the patients with skin lesions; 73% of patients with MEN 2A had these skin lesions.

Histopathology. The lesions usually contain deposits of amorphous, amyloid-like material in the papillary dermis (Pacini et al. 1993; Kousseff 1995). The epidermis shows orthokeratotic hyperkeratosis, elongation of the rete ridges and rare apoptotic keratinocytes in the malpighian layer (Fig. 13.2) (Verga et al. 2003). Immune histochemical studies have shown amyloid that stained for keratin but not for calcitonin (Gagel et al. 1989).

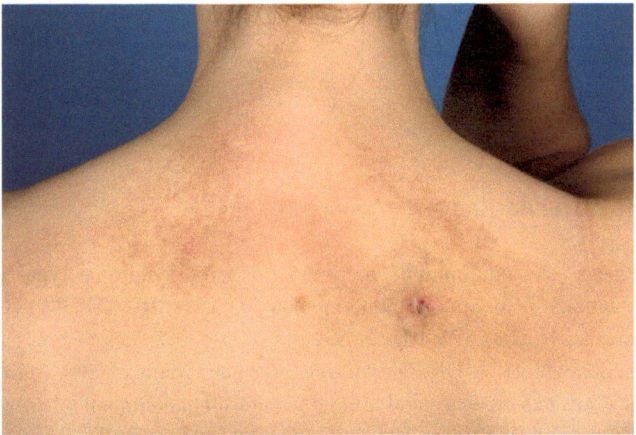

Fig. 13.1 Lichen amyloidosus in MEN 2A. In the intrascapular region, red-brownish agglomerated papules are observed; the area forms a heart-shaped figure. The larger skin defect on the left is the consequence of a biopsy. The 31-year-old patient was already operated on for thyroid carcinoma

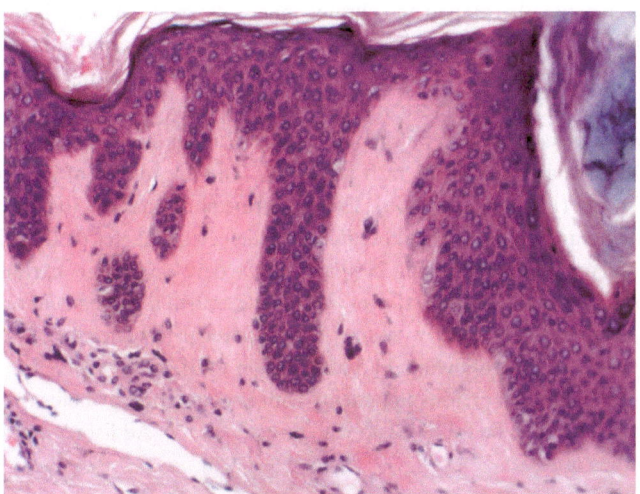

Fig. 13.2 Lichen amyloidosus, histopathology. There is hyperkeratotis, acanthosis and a necrotic keratinocyte. Small eosinophilic globules in the papillarly dermis can be hard to recognize in hematoxylin and eosin

Treatment. There is no standard treatment. Reports on treatment of LA with antihistamines, intralesional injection of glucocorticoids, etretinate, UVB irradiation and dermabrasion are available in the literature. Ten patients in the study of Ozkaya-Bayazit et al. (1997) were treated with DMSO, nine of them showed marked clinical improvement within a

13

few weeks. de Argila et al. (1996) and Verga et al. (2003) administered topical capsaicin 0.025%, but it was of limited success.

13.2
Autoimmune Polyendocrinopathy Syndrome Type I

Aetiopathogenesis. The autoimmune polyendocrinopathy syndrome type I (APS 1) is caused by mutations in the autoimmune regulator gene (AIRE, 240300) (OMIM). The gene map locus is 21q22.3. APS 1 has a penetrance of 100%, lack of preponderance and lack of association with HLA-DR (Obermayer-Straub and Manns 1998). Autosomal recessive inheritance was described several times, but autosomal dominant inheritance was also observed (Coleman and Hay 1997). The AIRE gene influences induction of self-tolerance. In APS type 1 the gene defect leads to the development of auto-antibodies against endocrine and other epithelial tissues, which induce autoimmune diseases. There are also antibodies neutralising IFNα and IFNo. The phenomenon may explain the disposition to infections in AIE, but it does not explain the predominance of candida infections (Meager et al. 2006).

APS 1 is characterized by the presence of two of three major clinical symptoms: Addison's disease, hypoparathyroidism and chronic mucocutaneous candidiasis (CMC). APS 1 exhibits highly variable symptoms including several other endocrinopathies and autoimmune diseases. Among 91 Finnish patients CMC existed in 60% of the patients, hypoparathyroidism in 32% and adrenocortical failure in 5%. Twenty-three percent of the patients had one to six other components before the diagnostic dyad: hepatitis, keratoconjunctivitis, chronic diarrhoea and periodic rash with fever. The prevalence of most components increased with age (Perheentupa 2006). The endocrine abnormalities may occur only late in lifetime and progress slowly. Suzuki et al. (2004) detected diabetes mellitus in a 58-year-old woman, and only in the following 20 years did she develop vitiligo, chronic thyroiditis and pernicious anaemia. Hunger-Dathe et al. 2005 described a 34-year-old male suffering from hypogonadism and general weakness due to adrenal insufficiency, who developed skin features only in the following 11 years. Hügle et al. (2004) underlined that early colouration of palmar skin creases in patients with known type I diabetes mellitus should serve as a warning sign to be followed up with investigation of Addison's disease and other endocrinopathies of APS.

Cutaneous Manifestation. CMC is usually the first manifestation of APS 1 seen even in childhood (López-Jornet et al. 2005). It may include seborrhoic dermatitis, hyperkeratotic candidosis of the scalp and other areas, paronychia and onychomycosis, angulus infectiosus (Fig. 13.3), oral aphthae, conjunctivitis and blepharitis with chalazions. Other skin diseases are also observed. In the study of Collins et al. (2006), cutaneous manifestations of APS type I were documented in eighteen patients (seven males and 11 females) from 15 families in Ireland. All patients had evidence of CMC which was an early feature, often predating the diagnosis of APS (10/18 patients). 13 (72%) had candidal onychomycosis or paronychia, six (33%) had alopecia areata and two had vitiligo. There was no correlation between the type of AIRE mutations and the clinical presentation (Collins et al. 2006).

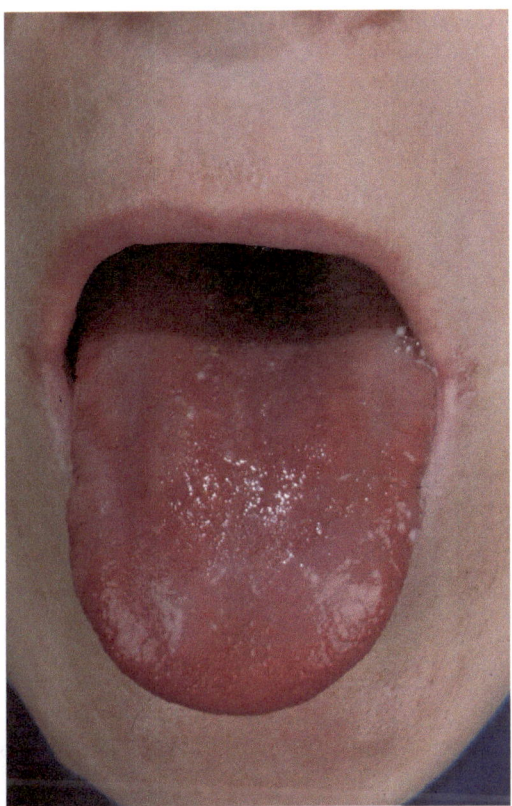

Fig. 13.3 APS type I, Chronic mucocutaneous candidosis. A 10-year-old boy with chronic angulus infectiosus and erosions of the tongue, in which candida albicans was demonstrable. Topical antimycotic treatment improved the lesions only for a short time

In rare cases, CMC may be absent in the syndrome. Bhansali et al. (2003) described a 16-year-old boy with APS type I, in whom chronic mucocutaneous candidiasis was absent. In our department we observed a patient born in 1986 for several years with APS 1, who showed hypoparathyroidism, adrenal insufficiency, hypogonadism with gynecomastia and pituitary delayed growth at the age of 16 years (Fig. 13.4). He was treated with vitamin D3, hydrocortisone and others. The hypogonadism was not treated; no pubertal development and body hair were demonstrable. As skin diseases, he showed alopecia areata totalis and vitiligo, but no CMC. Ten years earlier, the alopecia areata was less advanced (Fig. 13.5).

The typical autoimmune skin diseases observed in APS 1 are vitiligo and alopecia areata. The risk of alopecia areata is more than ten times higher in patients with APS than in healthy individuals. The study showed that the AIRE 961G allele is a potent risk factor (>3) for the development of severe alopecia areata (Tazi-Ahnini et al. 2002), but the two diseases frequently occur in patients without APS 1. Since the skin diseases are also frequent in patients without APS 1, it is highly questionable whether all patients demonstrat-

13

Fig. 13.4 APS 1. A 15-year-old
patient with hypogonadism including
gynecomastia showed alopecia areata
totalis and vitiligo, but no CMC

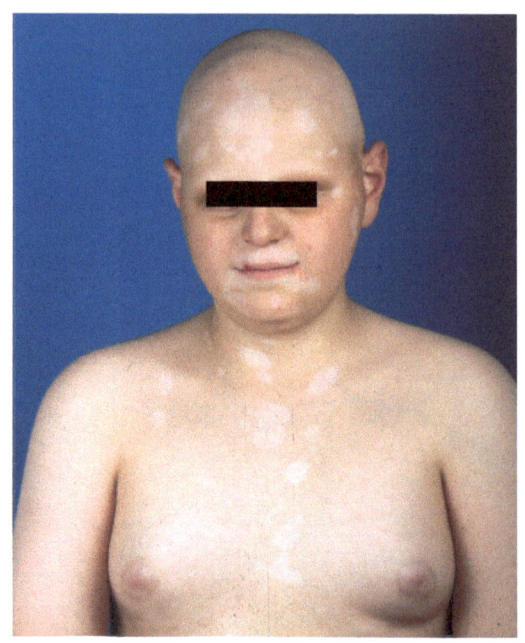

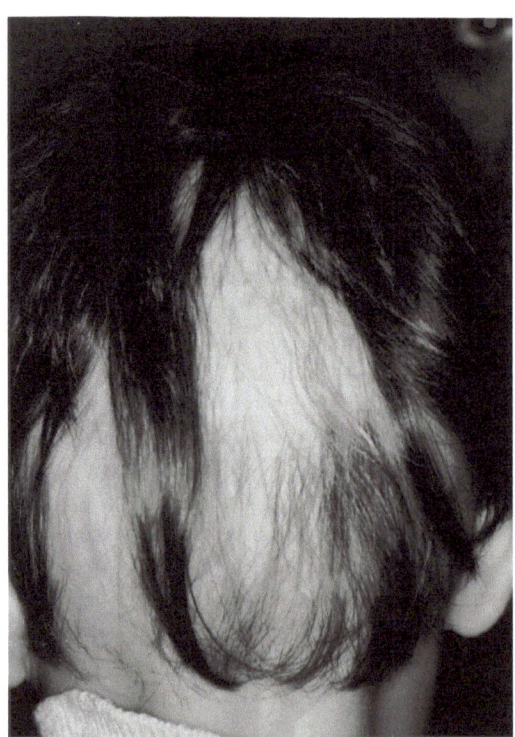

Fig. 13.5 APS 1. The same patient as
in Fig. 13.4 at the age of 2-years.
The alopecia areata is less advanced

ing vitiligo or alopecia areata should be assessed for other autoimmune diseases and APS 1 (Amerio et al. 2006).

Other skin lesions associated with APS 1, understandable on grounds of altered immune responses, have been described in case reports: A 45-year-old woman with known APS type I developed toxic epidermal necrolysis (TEN) and died within 10 days after onset. The authors suggested that some pathogenetic mechanisms of APS 1 are shared with TEN (Porzionato et al. 2004). Further, recurrent infection with herpes simplex virus type 1 (Nagafuchi et al. 2007), pigmented basal cell carcinoma (Sand et al. 2005), and condylomata acuminata in a 21-year-old woman (Oblinger et al. 1997) have been observed. A 31-year-old patient developed non-traumatic cutaneous ulcers on the forearms on the basis of a lupus erythematosus. Panniculitis and vasculitis were demonstrated by histological examination and a lupus-like immunoglobulin and complement-factor binding pattern were demonstrated by immune histology (Füchtenbusch et al. 2003).

Treatment. Treatment regimen in the syndrome refers to the singular symptoms, e.g. antimycotic treatment of candidosis. Systemic drugs have to be administered, as topical antimycotic treatment is usually ineffective.

References

Amerio P, Tracanna M, De Remigis P, Betterle C, Vianale L, Marra ME, Di Rollo D, Capizzi R, Feliciani C, Tulli A. Vitiligo associated with other autoimmune diseases: polyglandular autoimmune syndrome types 3B + C and 4. Clin Exp Dermatol. 2006;31(5):746–9.

Bhansali A, Kotwal N, Suresh V, Murlidharan R, Chattopadhyay A, Mathur K. Polyglandular autoimmune syndrome type 1 without chronic mucocutaneous candidiasis in a 16 year-old male. J Pediatr Endocrinol Metab. 2003;16(1):103–5.

Breathnach SM. Amyloid and amyloidosis. J Am Acad Dermatol. 1988;18(1 Pt 1):1–16.

Bugalho MJ, Limbert E, Sobrinho LG, Clode AL, Soares J, Nunes JF, Pereira MC, Santos MA. A kindred with multiple endocrine neoplasia type 2A associated with pruritic skin lesions. Cancer. 1992;70(11):2664–7.

Chabre O, Labat F, Pinel N, Berthod F, Tarel V, Bachelot I. Cutaneous lesion associated with multiple endocrine neoplasia type 2A: lichen amyloidosis or notalgia paresthetica? Henry Ford Hosp Med J. 1992a;40(3–4):245–8.

Coleman R, Hay RJ. Chronic mucocutaneous candidosis associated with hypothyroidism: a distinct syndrome? Br J Dermatol. 1997;136(1):24–9

Collins SM, Dominguez M, Ilmarinen T, Costigan C, Irvine AD. Dermatological manifestations of autoimmune polyendocrinopathy-candidiasis-ectodermal dystrophy syndrome. Br J Dermatol. 2006;154(6):1088–93.

de Argila D, Ortiz-Romero PL, Ortiz-Frutos J, Rodriguez-Peralto JL, Iglesias L. Cutaneous macular amyloidosis associated with multiple endocrine neoplasia 2A. Clin Exp Dermatol. 1996;21(4):313–4.

Donovan DT, Levy ML, Furst EJ, Alford BR, Wheeler T, Tschen JA, Gagel RF. Familial cutaneous lichen amyloidosis in association with multiple endocrine neoplasia type 2A: a new variant. Henry Ford Hosp Med J. 1989;37(3–4):147–50.

Füchtenbusch M, Vogel A, Achenbach P, Gummer M, Ziegler AG, Albert E, Standl E, Manns MP. Lupus-like panniculitis in a patient with autoimmune polyendocrinopathy-candidiasis-ectodermal dystrophy (APECED). Exp Clin Endocrinol Diabetes. 2003;111(5):288–93.

13

Gagel RF, Levy ML, Donovan DT, Alford BR, Wheeler T, Tschen JA. Multiple endocrine neoplasia type 2a associated with cutaneous lichen amyloidosis. Ann Intern Med. 1989;111(10):802–6.

Gullu S, Gursoy A, Erdogan MF, Dizbaysak S, Erdogan G, Kamel N. Multiple endocrine neoplasia type 2A/localized cutaneous lichen amyloidosis associated with malignant pheochromocytoma and ganglioneuroma. J Endocrinol Invest. 2005;28(8):734–7.

Hügle B, Döllmann R, Keller E, Kiess W. Addison's crisis in adolescent patients with previously diagnosed diabetes mellitus as manifestation of polyglandular autoimmune syndrome type II– report of two patients. J Pediatr Endocrinol Metab. 2004;17(1):93–7.

Hunger-Dathe W, Braun A, Müller UA. Alopecia totalis, Hypotonie und erektile Dysfunktion bei einem 34-jährigen Mann. Schwierige Klärung einer gemeinsamen Ursache. Internist (Berl). 2005;46(6):690–4.

Jabbour SA, Davidovici BB, Wolf R. Rare syndromes. Clin Dermatol. 2006;24(4):299–316.

Kousseff BG. Multiple endocrine neoplasia 2 (MEN 2)/MEN 2A (Sipple syndrome). Dermatol Clin. 1995;13(1):91–7.

López-Jornet P, García-Ballesta C, Pérez-Lajarín L. Mucocutaneous candidiasis as first manifestation of autoimmune polyglandular syndrome type I. J Dent Child (Chic). 2005;72(1):21–4. abstr

Masu S, Hosokawa M, Seiji M. Amyloid in localized cutaneous amyloidosis: immunofluorescence studies with anti-keratin antiserum especially concerning the difference between systemic and localized cutaneous amyloidosis. Acta Derm Venereol. 1981;61(5):381–4.

Meager A, Visvalingam K, Peterson P, Möll K, Murumägi A, Krohn K, Eskelin P, Perheentupa J, Husebye E, Kadota Y, Willcox N. Anti-interferon autoantibodies in autoimmune polyendocrinopathy syndrome type 1. PLoS Med. 2006;3(7):e289.

Modigliani E, Cohen R, Campos JM, Conte-Devolx B, Maes B, Boneu A, Schlumberger M, Bigorgne JC, Dumontier P, Leclerc L, Corcuff B, Guilhem I. Prognostic factors for survival and for biochemical cure in medullary thyroid carcinoma: results in 899 patients. The GETC Study Group. Groupe d'étude des tumeurs à calcitonine. Clin Endocrinol (Oxf). 1998;48(3):265–73.

Nagafuchi S, Umene K, Yamanaka F, Oohashi S, Shindo M, Kurisaki H, Kudoh J, Shimizu N, Hara T, Harada M. Recurrent herpes simplex virus infection in a patient with autoimmune polyendocrinopathy-candidiasis-ectodermal dystrophy associated with L29P and IVS9–1G > C compound heterozygous autoimmune regulator gene mutations. J Intern Med. 2007;261(6):605–10.

Nunziata V, di Giovanni G, Lettera AM, D'Armiento M, Mancini M. Cutaneous lichen amyloidosis associated with multiple endocrine neoplasia type 2A. Henry Ford Hosp Med J. 1989;37(3–4):144–6.

Obermayer-Straub P, Manns MP. Autoimmune polyglandular syndromes. Baillieres Clin Gastroenterol. 1998;12(2):293–315.

Oblinger E, Cibis A, Peter RU, Proebstle TM. Genito-anale Condylomata acuminata, mukokutane Candidose, Vitiligo, Keratopathie und primärer Hypoparathyreoidismus bei autoimmunem polyglandulärem Syndrom Typ 1. Dtsch Med Wochenschr. 1997;122(45):1382–6

Ozkaya-Bayazit E, Baykal C, Kavak A. Lokale DMSO-Behandlung der makulösen und papulösen Amyloidose. Hautarzt. 1997;48(1):31–7.

Pacini F, Fugazzola L, Bevilacqua G, Viacava P, Nardini V, Martino E. Multiple endocrine neoplasia type 2A and cutaneous lichen amyloidosis: description of a new family. J Endocrinol Invest. 1993;16(4):295–6.

Perheentupa J. Autoimmune polyendocrinopathy-candidiasis-ectodermal dystrophy. J Clin Endocrinol Metab. 2006;91(8):2843–50.

Porzionato A, Zancaner S, Betterle C, Ferrara SD. Fatal toxic epidermal necrolysis in autoimmune polyglandular syndrome type I. J Endocrinol Invest. 2004;27(5):475–9.

Rivollier C, Emy P, Armingaud P, Buzacoux J, Chadenas D, Legoux A, Estève E. Notalgie paresthétique e néoplasie endocrinienne multiple de type IIA (syndrome de Sipple: 3 cas. Ann Dermatol Venereol. 1999;126(6–7):522–4.

Robinson MF, Furst EJ, Nunziata V, Brandi ML, Ferrer JP, Martins Bugalho MJ, di Giovanni G, Smith RJ, Donovan DT, Alford BR, et al. Characterization of the clinical features of five families with hereditary primary cutaneous lichen amyloidosis and multiple endocrine neoplasia type 2. Henry Ford Hosp Med J. 1992;40(3–4):249–52.

Salim T, Shenoi SD, Balachandran C, Mehta VR. Lichen amyloidosus: a study of clinical, histopathologic and immunofluorescence findings in 30 cases. Indian J Dermatol Venereol Leprol. 2005;71(3):166–9.

Sand M, Bechara FG, Sand D, Moussa G, Stücker M, Altmeyer P, Hoffmann K, Rotterdam S. Polyglandular autoimmune syndrome associated with pigmented basal cell carcinoma. J Dermatol. 2005;32(12):1044–7.

Suzuki C, Hirai Y, Terui K, Kohsaka A, Akagi T, Suda T. Slowly progressive type 1 diabetes mellitus associated with vitiligo vulgaris, chronic thyroiditis, and pernicious anemia. Intern Med. 2004;43(12):1183–5.

Tazi-Ahnini R, Cork MJ, Gawkrodger DJ, Birch MP, Wengraf D, McDonagh AJ, Messenger AG. Role of the autoimmune regulator (AIRE) gene in alopecia areata: strong association of a potentially functional AIRE polymorphism with alopecia universalis. Tissue Antigens. 2002;60(6):489–95.

Verga U, Fugazzola L, Cambiaghi S, Pritelli C, Alessi E, Cortelazzi D, Gangi E, Beck-Peccoz P. Frequent association between MEN 2A and cutaneous lichen amyloidosis. Clin Endocrinol (Oxf). 2003;59(2):156–61.

Weyers W, Weyers I, Bonczkowitz M, Diaz-Cascajo C, Schill WB. Lichen amyloidosus: a consequence of scratching. J Am Acad Dermatol. 1997;37(6):923–8.

Genetic Syndromes Including Endocrinopathies

14

Synopsis

NAME Syndrome (Carney Complex)

> Name syndrome is an autosomal dominant multiple neoplasia syndrome characterized by cardiac, endocrine, cutaneous and neural myxomatous tumours, as well as a variety of pigmented lesions of the skin and mucosae. It may simultaneously also involve multiple endocrine diseases such as primary pigmented nodular adrenocortical disease (some with Cushing's syndrome), pituitary adenoma, testicular neoplasms, thyroid adenoma or carcinoma and ovarian cysts.

POEMS Syndrome

> POEMS syndrome is an acronym composed of the cardinal features of polyneuropathy, organomegaly, endocrinopathy, M-protein and skin changes. The pathogenesis is unclear; there is no conspicuous heritability. An overproduction of vascular endothelial growth factor (VEGF) explains the microangiopathy, neovascularization and accelerated vasopermeability. Characteristic are glomeruloid hemangiomas. Treatment of POEMS syndrome requires invasive chemotherapy. Regimen including plasmapheresis, melphalan, prednisone and thalidomide was described.

McCune–Albright Syndrome

> McCune–Albright syndrome (polyostotic fibrous dysplasia) is a sporadic disease. Probably, the syndrome reflects mosaicism, resulting from a postzygotic mutation. The clinical features of the syndrome include polyostotic fibrous dysplasia, segmental café-au-lait macules and various primary endocrine abnormalities, such as thyroid hyperplasia, Cushing's syndrome, acromegaly and hyperprolactinemia, and hyperparathyroidism. The main disorder is precocious puberty in girls.

Neurofibromatosis Type 1

> Neurofibromatosis type 1 (NF1) is a frequent autosomal dominant genetic disorder. Various endocrine abnormalities have been found to be associated

Continued

Walter K. H. Krause, *Cutaneous Manifestations of Endocrine Diseases*,
DOI: 10.1007/978-3-540-88367-8, © Springer-Verlag Berlin Heidelberg 2009

14

Synopsis   *Continued*

with NF1; precocious puberty with growth defects is the most frequent one.
Another frequent endocrine abnormality is phaeochromocytoma. Diagnostic
criteria of NF1 are café-au-lait spots, neurofibromas, freckling, optic glioma,
Lisch nodules, bony lesion and a first-grade relative suffering from NF1. There
is no systemic treatment available. Neurofibromas may be excised for aesthetic
problems, freckling may be removed by Laser treatment.

14.1
NAME Syndrome (Carney Complex)

Aetiopathogenesis. Atherton et al. (1980) originally suggested the acronym NAME
syndrome for nevi, atrial myxoma, myxoid neurofibromata and ephelides as a designation
for the syndrome. Koopman and Happle (1991) suggested that the acronym NAME could
stand for nevi, atrial myxoma, mucinosis of the skin and endocrine overactivity. Later in
the literature, the term Carney complex (CNC; Carney et al. 1985) became accepted.

Name syndrome is an autosomal dominant multiple neoplasia syndrome characterized
by cardiac, endocrine, cutaneous and neural myxomatous tumours, as well as a variety
of pigmented lesions of the skin and mucosae. It may simultaneously also involve multiple endocrine glands, similar to classic multiple endocrine neoplasia syndromes 1 and 2
(OMIM). Carney complex type 1 is caused by mutation in the protein kinase A regulatory
subunit-1-alpha gene (PRKAR1A; 188830) on chromosome 17q.

Endocrine disorders in Carney complex include primary pigmented nodular adrenocortical disease (some with Cushing's syndrome), pituitary adenoma, testicular neoplasms,
thyroid adenoma or carcinoma and ovarian cysts. In rare cases, psammomatous melanotic
schwannoma, breast ductal adenoma and osteochondromyxoma may be present (Jabbour
et al. 2006).

Cutaneous Manifestations. The cutaneous features include: multiple lentigines in the face
and the eyelid of particular shape ('ink spot lentigines', Fig. 14.1), lentigines in the lips,
the oral cavity and in the genitoanal region; cutaneous myxoma (Fig. 14.2) and myxoid
neurofibromas on the face and the upper trunk and multiple freckles; as a differential diagnosis to neurofibromatosis, café-au-lait spots were absent. Among 338 patients worldwide,
the following clinical manifestations were recorded: spotty skin pigmentation in 77%,
cardiac myxoma in 53%, skin myxoma in 33%, pigmented nodular adrenocortical disease
(26%), and testicular neoplasms in 33% of male patients (Jabbour et al. 2006).

Histopathology. In the lentigines the epidermis is acanthotic with regularly elongated
rete ridges with basal hyperpigmentation. The basal layer shows an increase of singular
melanocytes. Sparse lymphohistiocytic infiltrates and melanophages in the papillary
dermis are common.

Cutaneous myxomas are hypocellular, well delineated tumours located in the dermis or
subcutis. They consist of bland, stellate and spindle shaped cells with vesicular nuclei set

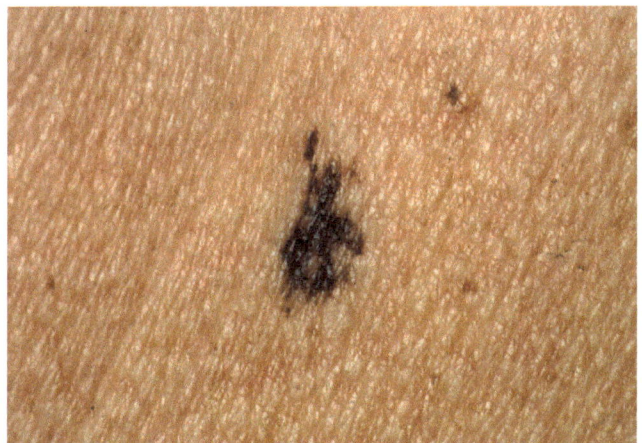

Fig. 14.1 Ink-spot lentigo in NAME syndrome. Flat, dark-brown pigmented area with irregular, bizarre border

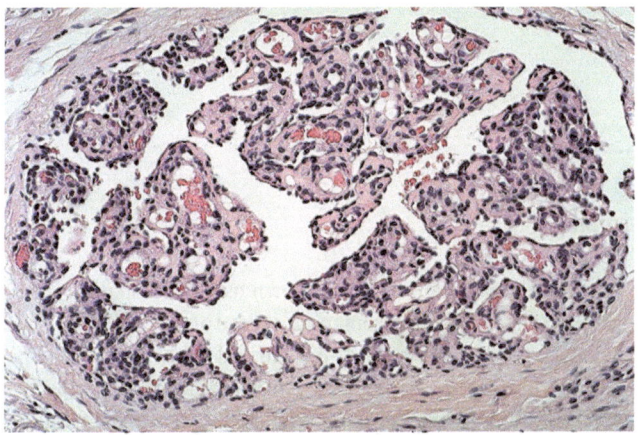

Fig. 14.2 Cutaneous myxomas in NAME syndrome. Cerebriform, skin-coloured soft tumour on the eyelid (Courtesy of Prof. R. Happle, Marburg)

in a myxoid pattern. They contain abundant small thin-walled vessels and mast cells. As epithelial components, they occasionally contain keratinous cysts or focal basaloid buds (Ferreiro and Carney 1994).

Epitheloid blue nevus has been observed as a rare variant of the blue nevus (Fig. 14.3). The epitheloid blue nevus is poorly demarcated, it is dome or wedge shaped and extends into the subcutaneous fat. It is composed of intensely pigmented globular and fusiform cells with small vesicular nuclei and prominent nucleoli. These are admixed with lightly pigmented spindle and dendritic cells. Mild cytological atypia occur, but mitotic figures are rare. The cells are arranged singularly or as fascicles among the collagen bundles.

Fig. 14.3 Blue nevus, in NAME syndrome, histopathology. The epitheloid blue nevus is poorly demarcated, it is dome or wedge shaped and extends into the subcutaneous fat. It is composed of intensely pigmented globular and fusiform cells with small vesicular nuclei and prominent nucleoli

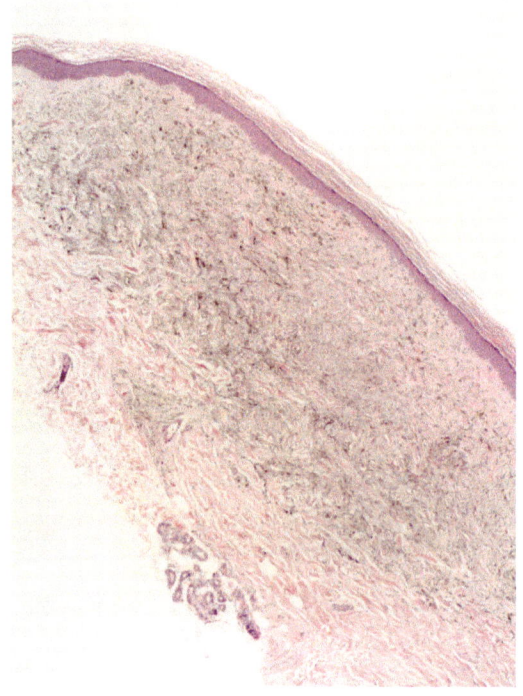

14.2
POEMS Syndrome

Aetiopathogenesis POEMS syndrome, also known as Crow–Fukase syndrome, is a rare multisystem disorder. The term is an acronym composed of the cardinal features of polyneuropathy, organomegaly, endocrinopathy, M-protein and skin changes. The pathogenesis is unclear; there is no conspicuous heritability. An overproduction of vascular endothelial growth factor (VEGF) to explain the microangiopathy, neovascularization and accelerated vasopermeability that occur in this syndrome was suggested (OMIM, +192240). The syndrome was predominantly observed in Asians, but it was also described in Caucasians (Longo et al. 1999). The most common endocrine abnormality in POEMS syndrome is hypogonadism, resulting in impotence (Amichai et al. 1994). Serologically, elevated levels of the proinflammatory cytokines interleukin-1, interleukin-6, tumour necrosis factor β, and VEGF are regularly found (Hudnall et al. 2003).

Cutaneous Manifestations. Characteristic are glomeruloid hemangiomas, which are probably due to overproduction of VEGF. The hemangiomas are multifocal vascular lesions, occurring in middle aged individuals on the trunk and proximal parts of the limbs (Fig. 14.4). In POEMS syndrome, 26–44% of patients show glomuleroid haemangiomas that may precede the diagnosis of the syndrome. Their detection is highly suggestive of POEMS syndrome. They have occasionally been observed in association with cryoglobulinemia, cold agglutination syndrome and monoclonal gammopathies of other origin (Velez et al.

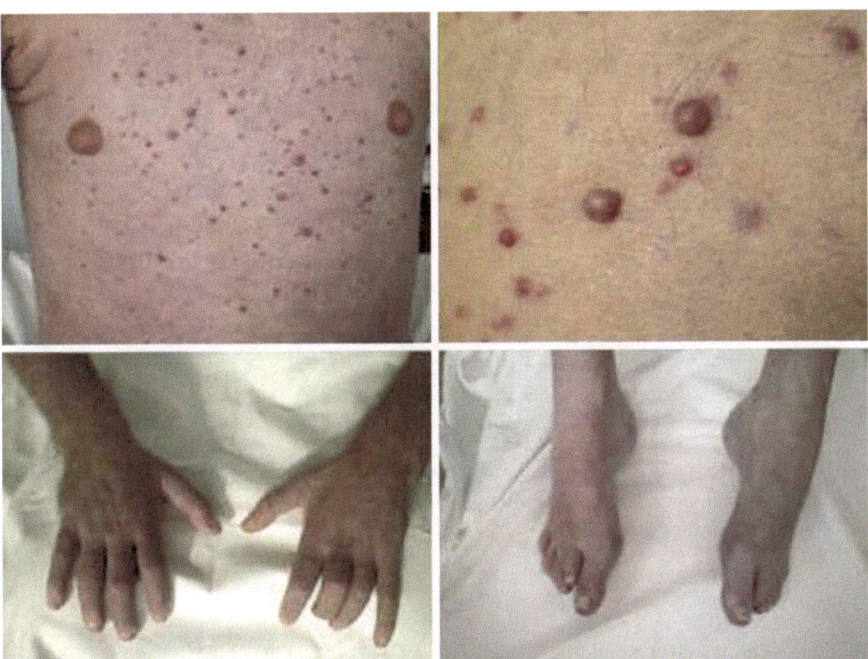

Fig. 14.4 POEMS syndrome. A 39-year-old Caucasian male shows glomeruloid haemangiomas together with polyneuropathy, organomegaly, endocrine dysfunctions and monoclonal gammopathy (from Longo et al. 1999, with permission)

2005; Granel et al. 2006; Ferran and Gimenez-Arnau 2006). Other skin changes include hyperpigmentation, hypertrichosis, skin thickening and digital clubbing (Hudnall et al. 2003). In a single case of POEMS syndrome a 59-year-old man showed progressive alopecia on the abdomen and the extensor surface of the thighs. The skin in these areas appeared to be otherwise normal (Amichai et al. 1994). An accompanying lymphadenopathy is often suggestive of Castleman disease (angiofollicular lymphoid hyperplasia), associated with human herpesvirus 8 (Hudnall et al. 2003). Serologically, elevated levels of the proinflammatory cytokines interleukin-1, interleukin-6, tumour necrosis factor β, and vascular endothelial growth factor are regularly found (Hudnall et al. 2003).

Histopathology. The glomeruloid hemangiomas show several dilated vascular spaces containing groups of irregular aggregates of capillary loops surrounded by pericytes (Fig. 14.5). The structures resemble renal glomeruli. The vascular spaces are lined by a single layer of plump stromal cells with the immune histochemical profile of endothelial cells, characterized by intracytoplasmatic vacuoles containing PAS-positive globules and surrounding pericytes. These cells probably represent immature elements that had accumulated immune globulins from the circulation (Chan et al. 1990; Ferran and Gimenez-Arnau 2006). As a cutaneous feature of the monoclonal plasmacytic proliferation appearing in POEMS syndrome cutaneous plasmocytosis may be present (Cerottini et al. 2001). Recently two types of cells with a different immunotype have been described (Kishimoto et al. 2000).

14

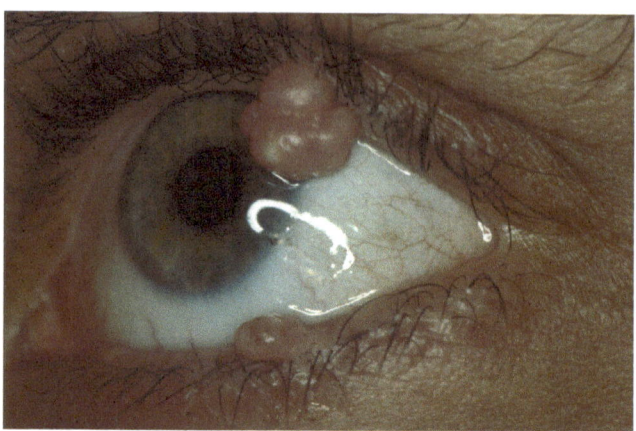

Fig. 14.5 POEMS syndrome, histopathology of glomeruloid hemangioma: A vascular space with intraluminal aggregates of capillary loops resembling renal glomeruli (Courtesy of Dr. Heinz Kutzner, Friedrichshafen)

While the capillary-type endothelial cells were CD31+, CD34+, UEAI+ and CD68−, the sinusoidal endothelial cells had a CD31+, CD34−, UEAI− and CD68+ phenotype.

The plasma cell proliferation of Castleman disease appears to be due to the actions of the HHV-8. An association of POEMS syndrome in general with HHV-8 has been suggested due to case reports demonstrating HHV-8 DNA sequences in the tissues circulating anti–HHV- 8 antibodies (Hudnall et al. 2003).

Treatment. Treatment of POEMS syndrome requires invasive chemotherapy. Because of the rarity of the syndrome, no controlled studies are available. Regimen including plasmapheresis, melphalan, prednisone and thalidomide was described (Longo et al. 1999; Sinisalo et al. 2004;Chan et al. 2006). A low-dose UVA1-treatment led to marked clinical improvement of cutaneous lesions (Schaller et al. 2001).

14.3
McCune–Albright Syndrome

Aetiopathogenesis. McCune–Albright syndrome (polyostotic fibrous dysplasia, 174800) is a sporadic disease, which is described twice as often in girls as in boys. It is usually caused by activating mutations in the GNAS1 gene (guanine nucleotide-binding protein, alpha-stimulating activity polypeptide 1). Guanine nucleotide-binding proteins (G proteins) transduce extracellular signals received by transmembrane receptors to effector proteins. The activity of hormone-sensitive adenylate cyclase is regulated by at least two G proteins, one stimulatory (Gs) and one inhibitory. Each G protein is a heterotrimer composed of an alpha, beta and gamma subunit. The GNAS1 gene encodes the alpha subunit of the G stimulatory protein. Gene map locus is 20q13.2 (OMIM).

Happle (1986) suggested that the syndrome reflects mosaicism, resulting from a postzygotic mutation, which is why the disorder always occurs sporadically. This was subsequently proven by demonstration of the mutation in peripheral blood leukocytes but not in DNA from cells of clinically normal skin.

The clinical features of the syndrome include polyostotic fibrous dysplasia, segmental café-au-lait macules and various primary endocrine abnormalities, such as thyroid hyperplasia, Cushing's syndrome, acromegaly and hyperprolactinemia, and hyperparathyroidism. The main disorder is precocious puberty in girls, which may often begin in the first 2 years of life. This is due to the autonomously functioning luteinized follicular cysts, while the GnRH secretion pattern is prepuberal. Precocious puberty in boys is less conspicuous and this may explain why the disorder is described in girls more often than in boys.

Cutaneous Manifestations. These are café-au-lait spots of characteristic shape (Fig. 14.6). The pigment patches are large lesions with irregular margins (shaped like 'the coast of

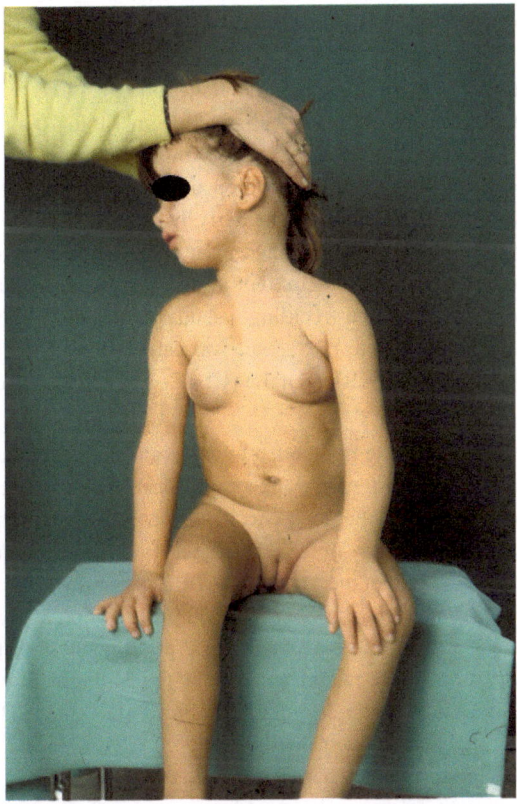

Fig. 14.6 McCune–Albright syndrome. Five-year-old girl with large pigment patches, which show irregular margins following the Blaschko lines and with precocious puberty. She had regular menses from the first year of life (Courtesy of Prof. R. Happle, Marburg)

Maine'). They follow the Blaschko lines and may be limited predominantly to one side, stopping sharply at the midline. In contrast to these lesions, the cafe-au-lait spots in neurofibromatosis are described as smaller, more regularly outlined and disseminated rather than segmentally arranged. Furthermore, axillary freckling and neurofibromas are absent in McCune–Albright syndrome.

Treatment. There is no specific treatment of the syndrome available, but therapeutic efforts are symptom-oriented.

14.4
Neurofibromatosis Type 1

Incidence. Neurofibromatosis type 1 (von Recklinghausen's disease, NF1, OMIM 162200) is an autosomal dominant genetic disorder. Approximately one-half of the cases are familial; the remainder are new mutations. Post-zygotic mutations were likewise observed. Neurofibromatosis type 2 is an autosomal dominant disorder predisposing to multiple neoplastic lesions. The pathognomonic findings are bilateral acoustic neuromas (schwannomas) (De Goede-Bolder et al. 2001; Jabbour et al. 2006).

Estimates of the prevalence of NF1 have ranged from 1.0 to 10.4 per 10,000 inhabitants depending on the population observed. The estimates at birth are unreliable, because the characteristic café-au-lait macules develop only in the first years of life and the neurofibromas become more frequent after puberty. In a German survey, a total of 152,819 children at the age of 6 years were examined during preschool examination. Diagnostic criteria for NF1 were found in 51 of them: 6 or more having café-au-lait-spots larger than 5 mm diameter, axillary or inguinal freckling, pseudarthrosis of the tibia, or history of a first-degree relative with NF1. Thus prevalence was calculated to 1 in 2996 (CI 1:2260–1: 3984). This is equivalent to a prevalence of 3.3 (CI 4.2–2.5) per 10,000 children (Lammert et al. 2005).

Aetiopathogenesis. The NF1 gene is encoded by 60 exons including a total size of 350 kb on chromosome 17q11.2. Known mutations range from single nucleotide substitution to large genomic rearrangements. The gene encodes for a 2,818 amino acid protein called neurofibromin of a molecular mass of 327 kDa. Neurofibromin is ubiquitous in the nervous system and may play a role in the regulation of Ras activity, which is an oncogene. In cell culture, NF1 + /– fibroblasts showed increased proliferation and collagen synthesis. Loss of neurofibromin results in Ras-dependent and phosphatidylinositol 3-kinase (PI3)-dependent hyperactivation of the rapamycin (mTOR) signaling pathway. Another signal transduction pathway involves protein kinase C (PKC) (De Goede-Bolder et al. 2001; Gottfried et al. 2006; Lee and Stephenson 2007).

Various endocrine abnormalities have been found to be associated with NF1. Precocious puberty with growth defects is the most frequent one; the feature is present in 30% of patients with NF1. The children grow normally until puberty, thereafter height velocity decreases. The most frequent cause is optic pathway tumours (Virdis et al. 2003). As a consequence about half of 28 patients showed short height as adults and only 50% of the

Table 14.1 Diagnostic criteria of neurofibromatosis type 1 of the American National Neurofibromatois Foundation Clinical Care Advisory Board (Gutman et al. 1997)

The patient should have two or more of the following:
1. Six of more café-au-lait spots of 0.5 cm diameter before puberty and 1.5 cm thereafter
2. Two or more neurofibromas or any type or 1 or more plexiform neurofibromas
3. Freckling in the axillae or groins
4. Optic glioma
5. Two or more Lisch nodules (benign iris hamartomas)
6. A distinctive bony lesion such as dysplasia of the sphenoid bone or dysplasia or thinning of long bone cortex
7. A first-grade relative suffering from NF1

28 patients attained an adult height that was appropriate for their respective target height (Carmi et al. 1999).

Another frequent endocrine abnormality is pheochromocytoma in 0.1–5.7% of patients (Erem et al. 2007; Kramer et al. 2007). Other abnormalities include Hashimoto's thyroiditis (Yalcin et al. 2006), hyperthyroidism (Sakane et al. 1997), hyperparathyroidism (Moiton et al. 2002), hypogonadism (Wang et al. 2004), bilateral testicular tumour (Kume et al. 2001), diabetes mellitus (Zaka-ur-Rab and Chopra 2005), pancreatic endocrine tumours (Fujisawa et al. 2002), and malignant somatostatinoma (Bettini et al. 2007).

1. Cutaneous: most common type (Fig. 14.8)
2. Subcutaneous: these lesions present as firm, tender nodules along the course of peripheral nerves. On palpation, they are described as feeling like a bag of worms (Fig. 14.9)
3. Nodular plexiform: nodular plexiform neurofibromas appear as complex clusters along proximal nerve roots and major nerves. They are similar to subcutaneous neurofibromas. They can cause vertebral erosion that may result in compression of the spinal cord
4. Diffuse plexiform: these lesions usually involve multiple nerve fascicles, with serpiginous growth and significant vascularity, rendering complete surgical resection extremely difficult, if not impossible

Cutaneous Manifestations. Diagnostic criteria of NF1 were published by the American National Neurofibromatois Foundation Clinical Care Advisory Board (Table 14.1). The hallmarks of NF1 are the multiple café-ut-lait spots and cutaneous neurofibromas (Jabbour et al. 2006). Café-au-lait spots are flat, uniformly hyperpigmented macules of light brown colour (Fig. 14.7). They appear during the first year of age, their number increases during early childhood. Children with no other features of NF1 should be followed

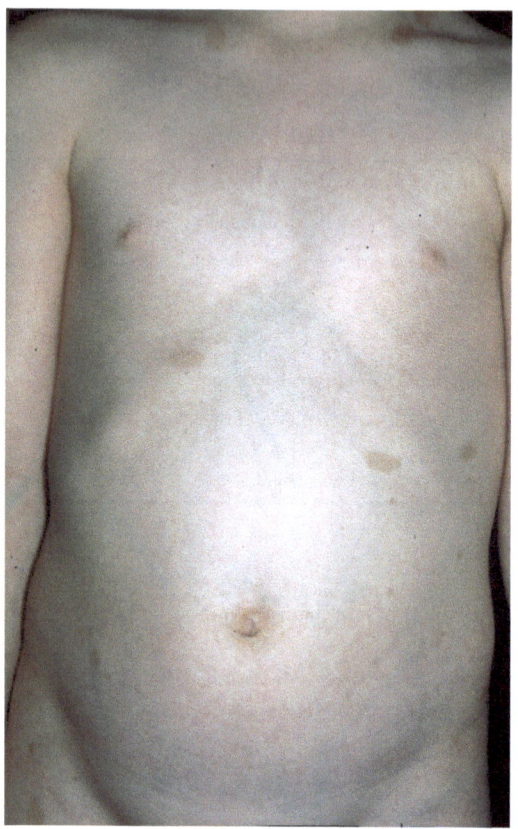

Fig 14.7 Neurofibromatosis type 1. Café-au-lait spots are flat, uniformly hyperpigmented macules of light brown colour, resembling white coffee. They tend to fade in later life, similar to the fading of pigmented nevi

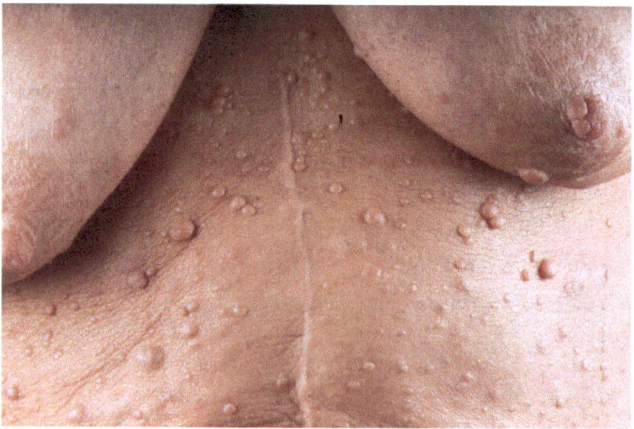

Fig. 14.8 Neurofibromatosis type 1. Neurofibromas are benign tumours, appearing as soft fleshy tumours, which can invaginate into the underlying dermal defect with light digital pressure ('button-holing'). This feature distinguishes them from other soft surface tumours. The number of tumours may vary from one to several hundreds

Fig. 14.9 Neurofibromatosis type 1. Subcutaneous neurofibromas present as firm, tender nodules along the course of peripheral nerves. On palpation, they feel like a 'bag of worms'

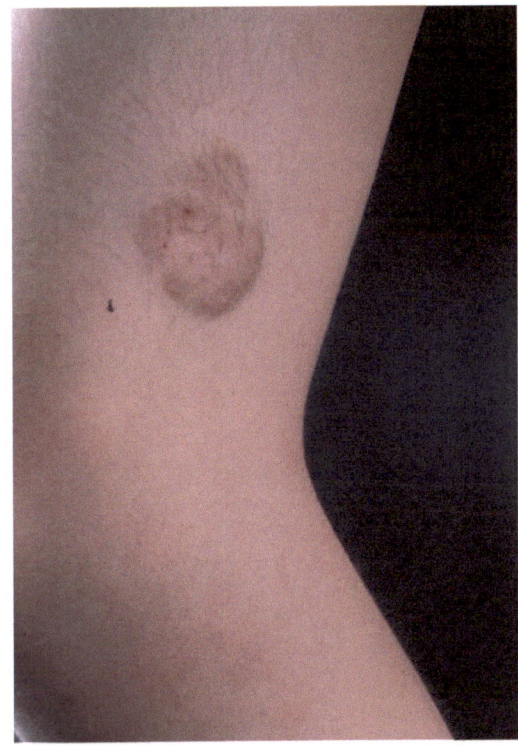

for several years for other clinical manifestations. 95% of adults with NF1 have café-au-lait spots. They tend to fade in later life, similar to the fading of pigmented nevi.

Neurofibromas are benign tumours that are composed of a mixture of Schwann cells, fibroblasts and mast cells. There are four types of neurofibromas:

The typical neurofibroma is a soft fleshy tumour, which can invaginate into the underlying dermal defect with light digital pressure ('button-holing'). This feature distinguishes them from other soft surface tumours. The tumours develop during adolescence and tend to increase in size and number with age and – in women – in particular during pregnancy, until they may have reached several hundreds of different size with the highest density over the trunk. They hold no risk of malignant development. However, they often represent a major cosmetic problem in adults (Jabbour et al. 2006).

Freckling occurs predominantly in the axillary and groin areas. Freckling usually is not apparent at birth but often appears during early childhood. It may also occur in later life in the neckline or inframammary folds (Fig. 14.10).

Neurofibromas are frequently associated with melanocytic nevi and melanocytic hyperplasia, which appears to be plausible, because the mutation that produces neurofibromatosis, also causes hyperplasia of Schwann cells, perineural fibroblasts and the normal components of neurofibromas and melanocytes (Ball and Kho 2005; De Schepper et al. 2005). Patients with NF1 develop benign and malignant tumours of the CNS and other

14

Fig. 14.10 Neurofibromatosis type 1. Freckling is an aggregation of light brown macules not exceeding 3 mm in size. It occurs mostly in the axillary and groin areas. Freckling usually is not apparent at birth but often appears during early childhood

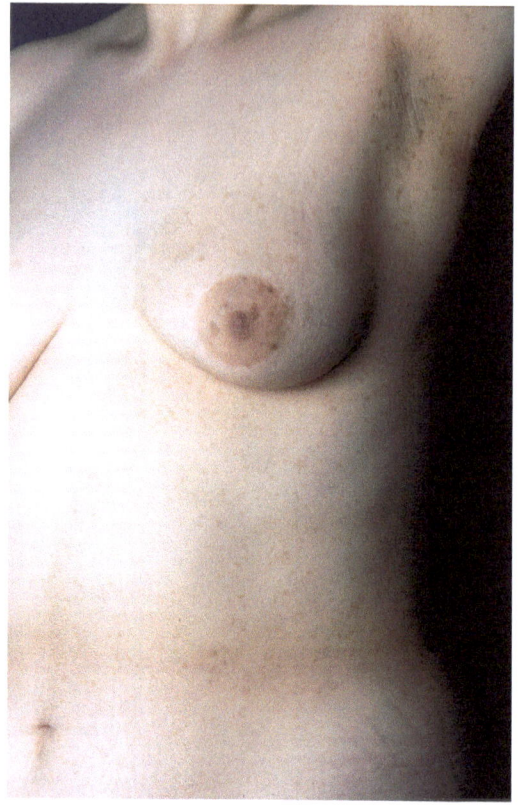

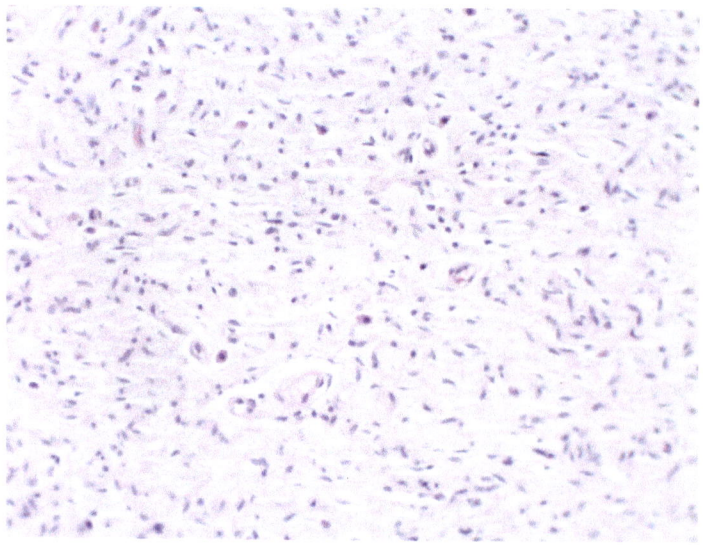

Fig. 14.11 Neurofibromatosis type 1, histopathology of neurofibroma: Small spindle cells with elongated, wavy nuclei and interdispersed mast cells

nerval tissues at increased frequency throughout life. The overall risk of malignancy in NF1 is estimated at 2–10% of affected individuals (Jabbour et al. 2006).

Lisch nodules are elevated, often pigmented small tumours of the iris. They remain asymptomatic throughout life. Bilateral Lisch nodules are highly characteristic for NF1 (Ceuterick et al. 2005).

Histopathology. Café-au-lait macules show hyperpigmentation of the basal keratinocytes, the number of melanocytes is increased, showing occasionally giant melanosomes. Cutaneous neurofibromas are well-defined, non-encapsulated tumours located in the dermis; they may extend into the subcutis. They consist of loosely arranged fascicles of spindle cells with scant, indefinite cytoplasm and elongated, wavy nuclei (Fig. 14.11). Histochemically immune, the cells stain positively for S100. The matrix is filled with abundant mucin and may be sclerosed or hyalinized. Blood vessels in the stroma and mast cells are proliferated. Plexiform neurofibroma are myxoid or fascicular enlargements of pre-existing nerves in the deep dermis or subcutis. They are embedded in a mucin-rich stroma in between delicate collagen bundles, fibroblasts and Schwann cells.

Treatment. There is no systemic treatment available. Neurofibromas may be excised for aesthetic problems, freckling may be removed by Laser treatment.

References

Amichai B, Giryes H, Ariad S, Grunwald MH, Halevy S. Alopecia as a rare cutaneous manifestation of POEMS syndrome. Br J Dermatol. 1994;131(2):297–8.

Atherton DJ, Pitcher DW, Wells RS, MacDonald DM. A syndrome of various cutaneous lesions, myxoid neurofibromata and atrial myxoma: the NAME syndrome. Br J Dermatol. 1980;103:421–9.

Ball NJ, Kho GT. Melanocytic nevi are associated with neurofibromas in neurofibromatosis, type I, but not sporadic neurofibromas: a study of 226 cases. J Cutan Pathol. 2005;32(8):523–32.

Bettini R, Falconi M, Crippa S, Capelli P, Boninsegna L, Pederzoli P. Ampullary somatostatinomas and jejunal gastrointestinal stromal tumor in a patient with Von Recklinghausen's disease. World J Gastroenterol. 2007;13(19):2761–3.

Carmi D, Shohat M, Metzker A, Dickerman Z. Growth, puberty, and endocrine functions in patients with sporadic or familial neurofibromatosis type 1: a longitudinal study. Pediatrics. 1999;103(6 Pt 1):1257–62.

Carney JA, Gordon H, Carpenter PC, Shenoy BV, Go VL. The complex of myxomas, spotty pigmentation, and endocrine overactivity. Medicine (Baltimore). 1985;64(4):270–83.

Cerottini JP, Guillod J, Vion B, Panizzon RG. Cutaneous plasmacytosis: an unusual presentation sharing features with POEMS syndrome? Dermatology. 2001;202(1):49–51.

Ceuterick SD, Van Den Ende JJ, Smets RM. Clinical and genetic significance of unilateral Lisch nodules. Bull Soc Belge Ophtalmol. 2005;(295):49–53.

Chan JK, Fletcher CD, Hicklin GA, Rosai J. Glomeruloid hemangioma. A distinctive cutaneous lesion of multicentric Castleman's disease associated with POEMS syndrome. Am J Surg Pathol. 1990;14(11):1036–46.

Chan PT, Lee KC, Chong LY, Lo KK, Cheung YF. Glomeruloid haemangioma with cerebriform morphology in a patient with POEMS syndrome. Clin Exp Dermatol. 2006;31(6):775–7.

de Goede-Bolder A, Cnossen MH, Dooijes D, van den Ouweland AM, Niermeijer MF. Van gen naar ziekte: neurofibromatosis type 1 [From gene to disease; neurofibromatosis type 1]. Ned Tijdschr Geneeskd. 2001;145(36):1736–8.

De Schepper S, Boucneau J, Lambert J, Messiaen L, Naeyaert JM. Pigment cell-related manifestations in neurofibromatosis type 1: an overview. Pigment Cell Res. 2005;18(1):13–24.

Erem C, Onder Ersöz H, Ukinç K, Hacihasanoglu A, Alhan E, Cobano lu U, Koçak M, Erdöl H. Neurofibromatosis type 1 associated with pheochromocytoma: a case report and a review of the literature. J Endocrinol Invest. 2007;30(1):59–64.

Ferran M, Gimenez-Arnau AM. Multiple eruptive angiomatous lesions in a patient with multiple myeloma. Glomeruloid hemangiomas associated with POEMS syndrome. Arch Dermatol. 2006;142(11):1501–6.

Ferreiro JA, Carney JA. Myxomas of the external ear and their significance. Am J Surg Pathol. 1994;18(3):274–80.

Fujisawa T, Osuga T, Maeda M, Sakamoto N, Maeda T, Sakaguchi K, Onishi Y, Toyoda M, Maeda H, Miyamoto K, Kawaraya N, Kusumoto C, Nishigami T. Malignant endocrine tumor of the pancreas associated with von Recklinghausen's disease. J Gastroenterol. 2002;37(1):59–67.

Gottfried ON, Viskochil DH, Fults DW, Couldwell WT. Molecular, genetic, and cellular pathogenesis of neurofibromas and surgical implications. Neurosurgery. 2006;58(1):1–16; discussion 1–16.

Granel B, Serratrice J, de Roux-Serratrice C, Ene N, Disdier P, Weiller PJ. Multiple cutaneous angiomas and Poems syndrome. Presse Med. 2006;35(3 Pt 1):430–2.

Gutmann DH, Aylsworth A, Carey JC, Korf B, Marks J, Pyeritz PE, et al. The diagnostic evaluation and multidisciplinary management of neurofibromatosis 1 and neurofibromatosis 2. JAMA. 1997;278:51–57

Happle R. The McCune-Albright syndrome: a lethal gene surviving by mosaicism. Clin Genet. 1986;29(4):321–4.

Hudnall SD, Chen T, Brown K, Angel T, Schwartz MR, Tyring SK. Human herpesvirus-8-positive microvenular hemangioma in POEMS syndrome. Arch Pathol Lab Med. 2003;127(8):1034–6

Jabbour SA, Davidovici BB, Wolf R. Rare syndromes. Clin. Dermatol. 2006;24(4):299–316.

Kishimoto S, Takenaka H, Shibagaki R, Noda Y, Yamamoto M, Yasuno H. Glomeruloid hemangioma in POEMS syndrome shows two different immunophenotypic endothelial cells. J Cutan Pathol. 2000;27(2):87–92.

Koopman RJJ, Happle R. Autosomal dominant transmission of the NAME syndrome (nevi, atrial myxoma, mucinosis of the skin and endocrine overactivity). Hum Genet. 1991;86:300–4.

Kramer K, Hasel C, Aschoff AJ, Henne-Bruns D, Wuerl P. Multiple gastrointestinal stromal tumors and bilateral pheochromocytoma in neurofibromatosis. World J Gastroenterol. 2007;13(24):3384–7.

Kume H, Tachikawa T, Teramoto S, Isurugi K, Kitamura T. Bilateral testicular tumour in neurofibromatosis type 1. Lancet. 2001;357(9253):395–6.

Lammert M, Friedman JM, Kluwe L, Mautner VF. Prevalence of neurofibromatosis 1 in German children at elementary school enrollment. Arch Dermatol. 2005;141(1):71–4.

Lee MJ, Stephenson DA. Recent developments in neurofibromatosis type 1. Curr Opin Neurol. 2007;20(2):135–41.

Longo G, Emilia G, Torelli U. Skin changes in POEMS syndrome. Haematologica. 1999;84:86

Moiton MP, Bijou F, Vargas F, Valentino R, Gruson D, Hilbert G, Bénissan G, Cardinaud JP. Association of type 1 neurofibromatosis and primary hyperparathyroidism. Presse Med. 2002;31(34):1604–5.

Sakane N, Shirakata S, Jin MB, Torii T, Yoshida T. von Recklinghausen's disease with hyperthyroidism. Intern Med. 1997;36(12):938.

Schaller M, Romiti R, Wollenberg A, Prinz B, Woerle B. Improvement of cutaneous manifestations in POEMS syndrome after UVA1 phototherapy. J Am Acad Dermatol. 2001;45(6): 969–70.

Sinisalo M, Hietaharju A, Sauranen J, Wirta O. Thalidomide in POEMS syndrome: case report. Am J Hematol. 2004;76(1):66–8.

Velez D, Delgado-Jimenez Y, Fraga J. Solitary glomeruloid haemangioma without POEMS syndrome. J Cutan Pathol. 2005;32(6):449–52.

Virdis R, Street ME, Bandello MA, Tripodi C, Donadio A, Villani AR, Cagozzi L, Garavelli L, Bernasconi S. Growth and pubertal disorders in neurofibromatosis type 1. J Pediatr Endocrinol Metab. 2003;16(Suppl 2):289–92.

Wang CY, Young C, Chu LW, Tsai WY. Hypopituitarism associated with neurofibromatosis type 1: report of one case. Acta Paediatr Taiwan. 2004;45(1):48–51.

Yalcin B, Tamer E, Gür G, Oztas P, Polat MU, Alli N. Neurofibromatosis 1/Noonan syndrome associated with Hashimoto's thyroiditis and vitiligo. Acta Derm Venereol. 2006;86(1):80–1.

Zaka-ur-Rab Z, Chopra K. Diabetes melliitus in neurofibromatosis I: an unusual presentation. Indian Pediatr. 2005;42(2):185–6.

Endocrine Cells of the Skin

15

Synopsis

Merkel Cell Carcinoma

> Merkel cell carcinoma (MCC) is a highly aggressive malignant tumour, origi-
> nating from the Merkel cells as endocrine cells of the skin, which are normal
> constituents of the epidermis. The majority of patients with MCC are older than
> 65 years of age; immunosuppression and ultraviolet irradiation are risk factors.
> Histopathologically, the tumour is composed of small blue cells with round-
> to-oval, hyperchromatic nuclei and scant cytoplasm, which resemble bronchial
> small cell carcinoma. For treatment, surgical intervention and additional radia-
> tion of the tumour site including the associated lymph nodes is recommended. If
> distant metastases are present, chemotherapy should be performed. The progno-
> sis is poor; a 5-year-survival rate has been quoted from 30 to 75%.

15.1
Merkel Cell Carcinoma

Aetiopathogenesis. Merkel cells as endocrine cells of the skin are normal constituents of the
epidermis, and exist in considerable numbers in connection to the hair follicles and to the
Haarscheiben. They are hard to identify in a hematoxilin–eosin stained skin section. Their
specific appearance is observed by electron microscopy, in which the cells show neurosecre-
tory granules. These granules contain neuropeptides and biogenic amines, which denominate
these cells as neuroendocrine cells. In the cytoskeleton, Merkel cells express cytokeratins
of low-molecular weight (CK 8, 18, 19, 20). In particular CK20 and CK 18 are specific
markers for the cutaneous Merkel cell and can be used to visualize the cells. The intermediate filaments of the cytoskeleton are more loosely distributed than in keratinocytes. Merkel
cells express neuroendocrine markers including a structural protein characteristic of nerve

Walter K. H. Krause, *Cutaneous Manifestations of Endocrine Diseases*,
DOI: 10.1007/978-3-540-88367-8, © Springer-Verlag Berlin Heidelberg 2009

15

cells and chromogranin A in the secretory granules. Therefore the Merkel cell has also been considered to be a member of the amine precursor uptake and the decarboxylation (APUD) system. This suggestion was supported by the observation of synchronous somatostatinoma associated with Merkel cells, which might present a previously un-described neuroendocrine tumour syndrome (Fincher et al. 1999). A specific endocrine product of the Merkel cells, however, could not be identified till today (Moll and Moll 1992).

The origin of Merkel cells is not quite clear. One hypothesis suggests that they originate from the neural crest; the other, that they are modified keratinocytes, undergoing neuroendocrine differentiation in the epidermis (Lucarz and Brand 2007). The latter hypothesis is more widely accepted. Merkel cells appear as early as in the 7th–9th foetal week, being localized above the basal layer and expressing the specific CK20. This observation makes it plausible that they originate from embryonic basal keratinocytes (Moll et al., 2005).

As a function of Merkel cells, the action as a mechanoreceptor is established. Their association to the bulge region of the hair follicles may suggest paracrine trophic functions during hair regrowth. Their intimate contact with the Langerhans cells also argues for a functional role in the neuroimmunological system of the skin. Merkel cells may have dual functions, storing both local hormones and neurotransmitters.

Reasons for malignant transformation of Merkel cells are unclear. The risk is severely increased by immunosuppression and ultraviolet radiation. Most recent results suggest that a previously unknown polyomavirus, the Merkel cell polyomavirus (MCV) may play a role (Feng et al. 2008).

Cutaneous Manifestations. Merkel cell carcinoma (MCC) is a highly aggressive malignant tumour, giving rise to metastasis in lymph nodes and distant organs in most cases.

The incidence of MCC is estimated as 0.2–0.3/100,000 per year. The age-adjusted incidence rate of MCC increased from 0.15 per 100,000 in 1986 to 0.44 per 100,000 in 2001. The annual increase is higher than in melanoma during this period. The majority of patients are older than 65 years of age, there is a slight male preponderance (Bichakjian et al. 2007). In a study of Dancey et al. (2006) on 34 patients, MCC occurred predominantly in Caucasians (97%) with a mean age of 75 years. Most tumours have been located on the extremity; at diagnosis they had a mean size of 2.1 cm. 37% of the patients additionally had a previous history of squamous cell carcinoma of the skin, 18% of basal cell carcinoma and 20% of actinic keratosis. Ten percent of patients showed evidence of immune deficiency.

MCC evolves nearly exclusively in sun-exposed areas (Weisser et al. 2007) and patients treated with UV-A for psoriasis have a much higher prevalence for MCC than untreated patients (Bichakjian et al. 2007). Since MCC has been frequently described in association with squamous cells carcinoma, the possibility of differentiating this tumour from Merkel cells is suggested (Foschini and Eusebi 2000).

Several cases of MCC associated with iatrogenic immunosuppression (for transplantation or for tumour diseases) and with HIV infection have been reported. The patients also are at a younger age (Bichakjian et al. 2007; Veness and Harris 2007).

Due to its rarenes, MCC is rarely diagnosed at the time of first presentation. Typically, MCC presents as a blue or red, firm, nontender, solitary, dome-shaped nodule (Fig. 15.1). Tumours may have an unspecific, plaque-like appearance (Fig. 15.2) or may present as a subcutaneous mass. The overlying skin is mostly intact, but it may also be ulcerated

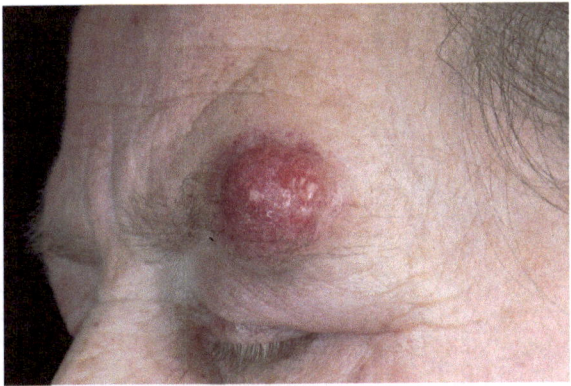

Fig. 15.1 Merkel cell carcinoma. A red, firm, nontender, solitary, dome-shaped nodule arises on the forehead

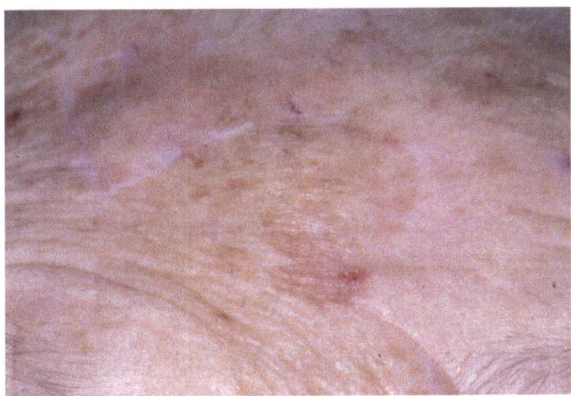

Fig. 15.2 Merkel cell carcinoma. Tumours may also have a plaque-like, unspecific appearance; a diagnosis without histopathological examination is impossible

(Bichakjian et al. 2007). Frequently, the tumour may be surrounded by small satellite tumours (Swann and Yoon 2007).

The differential diagnosis to squamous cell carcinoma of the skin, to lymphoma, or metastases from other tumors is not possible without histopathologic examination (Weisser et al. 2007)

For staging, a modified 4-tiered system is used: stage I patients with localized disease and tumor dimension < 2 cm, stage II localized disease, primary tumor dimension > 2 cm, stage III patients with regional disease, stage IV distant metastatic disease. This classification is consistent with the staging system of the AJCC (American Joint Committee on Cancer) (Bichakjian et al. 2007). About 30% of the patients show lymph metastases at the time of diagnosis, 10% also show distant metastases (Weisser et al. 2007). Maza et al. 2006 found Lymph node metastasis in 11 of 23 patients at the time of diagnosis.

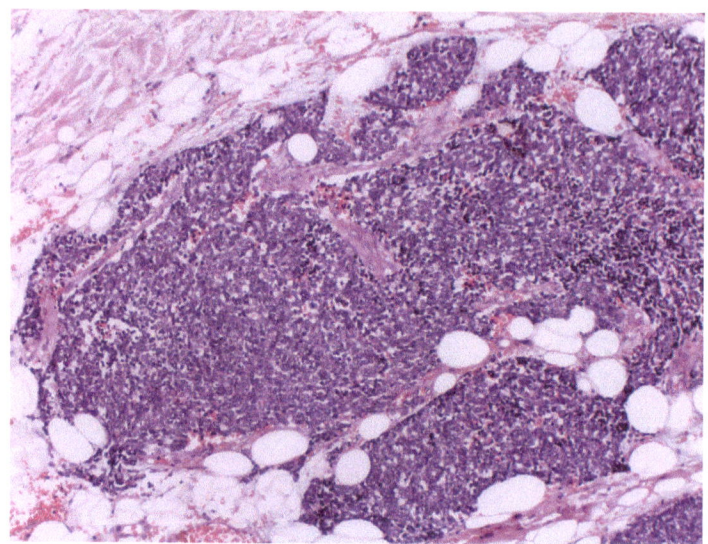

Fig. 15.3 Merkel cell carcinoma, histopathology. The overlying epidermis is primarily not involved. The tumor is composed of small blue cells with round-to-oval, hyperchromatic nuclei and scant cytoplasm. The nuclei have evenly dispersed, peppered chromatin

A sentinel lymph node excision was performed in eight patients. Recurrence developed in seven patients, only two of them had positive sentinel lymph nodes. The authors suggest that, although sentinel lymph node analysis is valuable for staging, the role in the prognosis is not fully elucidated.

Histopathology. MCC appears as a dermal tumour with infiltration of the subcutaneous fat. The overlying epidermis is primarily not involved. The tumour is composed of small blue cells with round-to-oval, hyperchromatic nuclei and scant cytoplasm (Fig. 15.3). The nuclei have evenly dispersed, peppered chromatin and inconspicuous nucleoli. Frequently, vascular invasion (31–60%), tumor necrosis (48–60%), perineural invasion (48%), and high mitotic rate have been observed. The epidermis is involved in 5–30% of tumours. Three types of tumour cells may be differentiated: the intermediate variant (about 50% of cells), the small cell variant, which resembles bronchial small cell carcinoma and the trabecular variant (Bichakjian et al. 2007).

The accurate diagnose of MCC by conventional light microscopic methods is challenging, but electron microscopy and immune histochemistry may be necessary (Swann and Yoon, 2007). Histochemically immune, the staining with antibodies to CK-20 is highly specific, but it was also positive in 33% of small cell lung cancer. An instrument for discrimination is thyroid transcription factor-1, which is consistently absent in MCC. Other markers with a high sensitivity for MCC included neuron-specific enolase and chromogranin A, synaptophysin (Bichakjian et al. 2007). Low levels of neuroendocrine differentiation in MCC have been associated with poor prognosis (Koljonen et al. 2005).

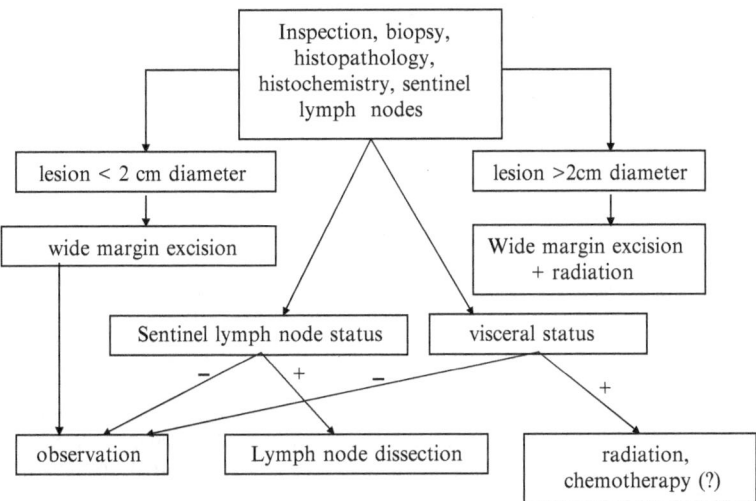

Fig. 15.4 Flow chart summarizing diagnosis and treatment schedules of MCC as proposed by Bichakjian et al. (2007)

Treatment. No guidelines are available for treatment. A flow chart summarizing diagnosis and treatment schedules was proposed by Bichakjian et al. (2007) (Fig. 15.4). As a primary treatment, surgical intervention is generally recommended, if lymphatic or distant metastases are absent. Excision should be performed with a wide margin of 3 cm around the tumour. Surgical removal alone, however, cannot avoid relapses, thus additional radiation of the tumour site including the associated lymph nodes is recommended. If distant metastases are present, the local treatment is less important, but chemotherapy is recommended. The use of combinations of cyclophosphamide, methotrexate, fluorouracil and/ or cisplatin, ectoposide, doxorubicine and vincristine was reported in the literature, but controlled studies are missing. Also single reports of successful remissions after application of octretoide, α-interferon and rituximab are available in the literature. Small series have achieved initial response rates of 100%, but the median duration of response is only 8 months. The response rates of second-line and third-line chemotherapy decrease considerably. An impact on survival rate was not demonstrated. Since patients with MCC are mainly older than 65 years, the myelosuppressive toxicity of the antineoplastic drugs is a matter of concern (Bichakjian et al. 2007; Weisser et al. 2007).

The prognosis of MCC is poor. 5-year-survival rate has been quoted from 30 to 75%. The following characteristics indicate a worse prognosis: high mitotic activity in the tumour; endolymphatic distribution of tumour cells; tumour size >2 cm; localisation in head or neck; male gender. The disease stage was identified as the strongest predictor of survival (Bichakjian et al. 2007; Weisser et al. 2007). An improvement of the prognosis as a consequence of the treatment cannot be concluded until now from the reports.

References

Bichakjian CK, Lowe L, Lao CD, Sandler HM, Bradford CR, Johnson TM, Wong SL. Merkel cell carcinoma: critical review with guidelines for multidisciplinary management. Cancer. 2007;110(1):1–12.

Dancey AL, Rayatt SS, Soon C, Ilchshyn A, Brown I, Srivastava S. Merkel cell carcinoma: a report of 34 cases and literature review. J Plast Reconstr Aesthet Surg. 2006;59(12):1294–9.

Feng H, Shuda M, Chang Y, Moore PS. Clonal integration of a polyomavirus in human Merkel cell carcinoma. Science. 2008;319(5866):1096–100.

Fincher RK, Christensen ED, Tsuchida AM. Ampullary somatostatinoma in a patient with Merkel cell carcinoma. Am J Gastroenterol. 1999;94(7):1955–7.

Foschini MP, Eusebi V. Divergent differentiation in endocrine and nonendocrine tumors of the skin. Semin Diagn Pathol. 2000;17(2):162–8.

Koljonen V, Haglund C, Tukiainen E, Bohling T. Neuroendocrine differentiation in primary Merkel cell carcinoma – possible prognostic significance. Anticancer Res. 2005;25(2A):853–8.

Lucarz A, Brand G. Current considerations about Merkel cells. Eur J Cell Biol. 2007;86(5):243–51

Maza S, Trefzer U, Hofmann M, Schneider S, Voit C, Krössin T, Zander A, Audring H, Sterry W, Munz DL. Impact of sentinel lymph node biopsy in patients with Merkel cell carcinoma: results of a prospective study and review of the literature. Eur J Nucl Med Mol Imag. 2006;33(4):433–40.

Moll I, Moll R. Early development of human Merkel cells. Exp Dermatol. 1992;1(4):180–4.

Moll I, Roessler M, Brandner JM, Eispert AC, Houdek P, Moll R. Human Merkel cells–aspects of cell biology, distribution and functions. Eur J Cell Biol. 2005;84(2–3):259–71.

Swann MH, Yoon J. Merkel cell carcinoma. Semin Oncol. 2007;34(1):51–6.

Veness MJ, Harris D. Role of radiotherapy in the management of organ transplant recipients diagnosed with non-melanoma skin cancers. Australas Radiol. 2007;51(1):12–20.

Weisser H, Hartschuh W, Greiner A, Bischof M, Enk A, Helmbold P. Das Merkel cell-Karzinom – klinisch oft verkanntclinically. Dtsch Med Wochenschr. 2007;132(30):1581–6.

Index